Agnes Walker

Modelling the socioeconomic status to health link in Australia

D1797144

Agnes Walker

Modelling the socioeconomic status to health link in Australia

A dynamic microsimulation approach

LAP LAMBERT Academic Publishing

Impressum/Imprint (nur für Deutschland/ only for Germany)

Bibliografische Information der Deutschen Nationalbibliothek: Die Deutsche Nationalbibliothek verzeichnet diese Publikation in der Deutschen Nationalbibliografie; detaillierte bibliografische Daten sind im Internet über http://dnb.d-nb.de abrufbar.

Alle in diesem Buch genannten Marken und Produktnamen unterliegen warenzeichen-, marken- oder patentrechtlichem Schutz bzw. sind Warenzeichen oder eingetragene Warenzeichen der jeweiligen Inhaber. Die Wiedergabe von Marken, Produktnamen, Gebrauchsnamen, Handelsnamen, Warenbezeichnungen u.s.w. in diesem Werk berechtigt auch ohne besondere Kennzeichnung nicht zu der Annahme, dass solche Namen im Sinne der Warenzeichen- und Markenschutzgesetzgebung als frei zu betrachten wären und daher von jedermann benutzt werden dürften.

Coverbild: www.purestockx.com

Verlag: LAP LAMBERT Academic Publishing AG & Co. KG
Theodor-Heuss-Ring 26, 50668 Köln, Germany
Telefon: +49 681 3720-310, Telefax: +49 681 3720-3109, Email: info@lap-publishing.com
Zugl.: Canberra,Australian National University,Dissertation,2005

Herstellung in Deutschland:
Schaltungsdienst Lange o.H.G., Berlin
Books on Demand GmbH, Norderstedt
Reha GmbH, Saarbrücken
Amazon Distribution GmbH, Leipzig
ISBN: 978-3-8383-0030-6

Imprint (only for USA, GB)

Bibliographic information published by the Deutsche Nationalbibliothek: The Deutsche Nationalbibliothek lists this publication in the Deutsche Nationalbibliografie; detailed bibliographic data are available in the Internet at http://dnb.d-nb.de.

Any brand names and product names mentioned in this book are subject to trademark, brand or patent protection and are trademarks or registered trademarks of their respective holders. The use of brand names, product names, common names, trade names, product descriptions etc. even without a particular marking in this works is in no way to be construed to mean that such names may be regarded as unrestricted in respect of trademark and brand protection legislation and could thus be used by anyone.

Cover image: www.purestockx.com

Publisher:
LAP LAMBERT Academic Publishing AG & Co. KG
Theodor-Heuss-Ring 26, 50668 Köln, Germany
Phone: +49 681 3720-310, Fax: +49 681 3720-3109, Email: info@lap-publishing.com

Printed in the U.S.A.
Printed in the U.K. by (see last page)
ISBN: 978-3-8383-0030-6

Acknowledgements

The author wishes to thank Professor Niels Becker - 'Chair' of the PhD supervisory panel - for his unwavering commitment to this thesis over the five long years it took to complete; for the overall guidance he provided to the project; for his valuable contributions to our joint paper to be published in *Public Health* (Chapter 5); and to the methodologies used to model health state transitions (Chapter 8). The author is also grateful to Professor Ann Harding, Director, National Centre for Social and Economic Modelling (NATSEM) for making DYNAMOD available for this thesis. The helpful comments on an earlier draft of this thesis by Professors Niels Becker and Ann Harding, and by Dr Simon Kelly of NATSEM are gratefully acknowledged. Finally, help from David Pederson of the University of Canberra on the use of the SAS language for statistical analyses, and from Richard Percival and Dr Simon Kelly of NATSEM with C programming and the understanding of the technical details essential for running and modifying DYNAMOD, were much appreciated.

Contents

Definitions...x

Symbols (used in section 4.4) xi

Abbreviations xii

CHAPTER 1   OVERVIEW...1

1.1   Introduction...1
    1.1.1   Background...1
    1.1.2   Aims of thesis 3

1.2   Reasons for choosing dynamic microsimulation..4
    1.2.1   Background...4
    1.2.2   Reasons for choosing dynamic microsimulation 7

1.3   New modules as part of an existing model versus a stand-alone model.............9

1.4   The dynamic microsimulation model chosen 10

1.5   Steps involved in adding new modules to DYNAMOD 13
    1.5.1   Key elements of the enhanced model 14
    1.5.2   The main steps 16
    1.5.3   The programming effort...17

1.6   Questions the enhanced model may address 19

1.7   Outline of thesis...20

PART 1: DEVELOPMENT OF THE HEALTH_SES AND HEALTH STATE
TRANSITION MODULES...22

CHAPTER 2   RELEVANT FINDINGS FROM THE LITERATURE 23

2.1   Mortality based studies of the health-SES links 23

2.2   Intergenerational effects...25

2.3   Labour market effects 26

2.4   Causality 27

2.5   Life course approach 29

2.6   Other countries' dynamic microsimulation models 30

2.7   Discussion 35

CHAPTER 3   CHOICE OF DATA SOURCES 36

3.1   **Data requirements** 36

3.2   **The data sources considered** 36

3.3   **Suitability of the health and disability surveys** 39

3.4   **The data sources chosen** 42

CHAPTER 4   METHODOLOGY USED IN DEVELOPING THE HEALTH_SES
MODULE   44

4.1 Overview of the development of the Health_SES module 45

4.2   **Indicators of health status** 48
    4.2.1   Mortality 48
    4.2.2   Disability 49

4.3   **Key factors affecting family income** 50

4.4   **Estimating disability and mortality rates by SES** 53
    4.4.1   Equations for computing mortality rates: able-bodied and disabled 54
    4.4.2   Equations linking disability and mortality by SES 55
    4.4.3   Equations for deriving future mortality rates 58

4.5   **Conclusion** 62

CHAPTER 5   COMPARING GEOGRAPHIC-AREA-BASED AND INDIVIDUAL-
BASED SES INDICATORS 63

5.1   **Aims of analyses** 64

5.2   **Indicators of health and socioeconomic status** 65

5.3   **Do the three types of SES measures produce similar estimates of health
inequalities?** 67

5.4   **Are some SES indicators better predictors of a person being disabled than
others?** 67

5.5   **Results** 68
    5.5.1   Inequalities in health by SEIFA – Objective (a) 68
    5.5.2   Comparing the predictive ability by type of SES indicator – Objective (b) 72

5.6   **Discussion** 73

5.7   **Conclusions and possible future improvements** 74
    5.7.1   Conclusions 76
    5.7.2   Possible future improvements 76

5.8   **Choosing the SES indicators for DYNAMOD** 77

CHAPTER 6   PREPARING THE INPUT DATA ON MORTALITY AND
DISABILITY BY AGE, SEX AND SOCIOECONOMIC STATUS...........................79

6.1   Introduction...79

6.2   Mortality rates..80
    6.2.1   By SES quintiles 80
    6.2.2   Over time..82

6.3   Disability prevalence..84

6.4   Disability decrement rates...85

CHAPTER 7   MODELLING SOCIOECONOMIC STATUS FOR THE BASE
DATASET AND THE PROJECTION YEARS...86

7.1   Modelling socioeconomic status in the Base dataset.............................86

7.2   Modelling socioeconomic status in the simulation years......................87

CHAPTER 8   MODELLING HEALTH STATE TRANSITIONS 90

8.1   The available data..91

8.2   The health states modelled 93

8.3   Methodology for estimating health transition probabilities 93
    8.3.1   Assumptions 93
    8.3.2   Computing health transition probabilities..................................94

8.4   Implementation in the model...98
    8.4.1   Input data...98
    8.4.2   Implementation in the Base dataset 98

CHAPTER 9   VALIDATION..99

9.1   Disability in the original model...100

9.2   Disability in the enhanced model...101

CHAPTER 10   LIMITATIONS..105

10.1   Alignment procedures 105
    10.1.1   Alignment procedures in the literature.......................................106
    10.1.2   Alignment processes used in DYNAMOD......................................108

10.2   Stochastic variations in model outputs 110

10.3   Sensitivity testing 111

10.4   Multiple-module validation...112

PART 2: APPLICATIONS OF THE ENHANCED MODEL.................................113

CHAPTER 11   NARROWER HEALTH INEQUALITIES 114

11.1   Description of scenario and assumptions..**114**

11.2   Impact on the number of deaths...**115**

11.3   Impact on numbers disabled and on health care and disability pension expenditures **118**

11.4   Discussion **123**
   11.4.1   Comparisons with findings from earlier studies.............................124
   11.4.2   Possible future improvements 125

CHAPTER 12   HEALTH AND THE ABILITY OF OLDER AUSTRALIANS TO STAY IN THE LABOUR FORCE...127

12.1 Recent policy initiatives and future directions.....................................**127**

12.2 Aims..**129**

12.3   Modelling the employment status of 65-70 year olds...........................**129**
   12.3.1   Data and methodology..130
   12.3.2   Choice of variables in explaining work patterns 130
   12.3.3   Logistic regression for the probability of working 132
   12.3.4   Imputing of 'work' status in the main model 134
   12.3.5   Validation...135

12.4   Description of the Base case and Scenario simulations **135**

12.5   Results: health and employment of 45-54 year olds versus 65-70 year olds...**136**

12.6   Results: predicted population of 65-70 year olds and the proportion working   **139**

12.7   Results: earnings of 65-70 Year Olds..**141**

12.8   Results: expenditures on the age pension for 65-70 year olds **144**

12.9   Results: comparing the Base case and Scenario results **146**

12.10   Discussion **147**

PART 3: OVERALL CONCLUSIONS..150

CHAPTER 13   CONCLUSIONS AND POSSIBLE FUTURE DEVELOPMENTS   151

13.1   Conclusions..**151**
   13.1.1 PART 1: Modelling the links between health and socioeconomic status 151

13.1.2 PART 2: Applications of the enhanced model 155

13.2 Possible future developments **156**

REFERENCES 160

REFERENCES 160

APPENDICES 174

A1 DESCRIPTION OF DYNAMOD - ORIGINAL VERSION AND THE WEALTH MODULE 175

A1.1 Original version **175**

A1.2 The Wealth module **184**

A2 POSSIBLE DATA SOURCES 186

A2.1 National Health Surveys (1977, 1983, 1989 and 1995) **186**

A2.2 Australian Longitudinal Study of Ageing (ALSA) **188**

A2.3 Disability surveys **189**

A2.4 Mortality statistics **192**
A2.4.1 Causes of deaths (ABS) 192
A2.4.2 Mortality by age sex and socioeconomic status 192

A3 SOCIO-ECONOMIC INDEXES FOR AREAS (SEIFA) 194

A4 CHANGES IN MORTALITY PATTERNS BY AGE AND SEX, 1990-92 TO 1995-97 196

A5 CHANGES IN DISABILITY PREVALENCE BY AGE AND SEX, 1993 AND 1998 200

A6 DERIVING INCOME-BASED SES INDICATORS FROM THE 1998 DISABILITY SURVEY 202

A6.1 Creating the basic SAS dataset **203**

A6.2 Deriving family income and computing income quintiles **205**

A6.3 Example of SAS code: deriving income-based SES indicators **206**

A7 DEMOGRAPHIC, HEALTH, EMPLOYMENT AND RESIDENTIAL CHARACTERISTICS OF AUSTRALIANS, 1998 209

A7.1 Introduction..**209**

A7.2 Disability by age and sex **209**

A7.3 The disabled population by income..**211**

A7.4 The disabled population by labour force status and institutionalisation **212**

A7.5 Duration of main disabling condition and patterns of comorbidities.............**213**

A8   THE MODIFIED OECD EQUIVALENCE SCALE...216

A9 HEALTH AS A REASON FOR NOT LOOKING FOR WORK 217

A10   AGE STANDARDISATION ACROSS SES QUINTILES..........................219

A11   STANDARD ERRORS AND STATISTICAL SIGNIFICANCE.................221

A12   EXAMPLE OF C CODE – COMPUTING AND IMPUTING SOCIO-
ECONOMIC STATUS 222

List of Figures and Tables

Figure 1: Elements of the enhanced version of DYNAMOD   15

Figure 2: Probability of Australians aged 25–65 years dying, by sex and quintile of socioeconomic disadvantage, 1995–97   24

Figure 3: Spenders on prescribed drugs, per cent of the population by age group, 1993-94 and 1998-99   40

Figure 4: Proportion of population disabled and/or with long-term-illness, 1998   41

Figure 5: The links modelled between mortality and disability, by SES   46

Table 1: Multiple regressions of 'equivalent family income quintile' for persons aged 20 years or over, 1998   51

Figure 6: Proportion disabled by age and type of SES indicator*   69

Figure 7: Proportion disabled by type of SES indicator,* 1998   70

Table 2: Differences in the proportion disabled by age and type of socioeconomic status indicator, 1998   71

Table 3: Logistic regressions – SES indicators as predictors of disability   72

Figure 8: Age distribution within SES quintiles, Disability Survey, 1998   75

Figure 9: Mortality rates, external causes, males age, SEIFA quintiles, 1995-7   81

Figure 10: Mortality rates for men, non-external causes (ie the disabled population), by single years of age, 1990-92 and 1995-97   83

Figure 11: Disability prevalence, males, by age, 1993 and 1998   84

Figure 12: Per cent of the population by age and health status, 1998   92

Table 4: Matrix algebra equations for transition probabilities - general notation   95

Table 5: Matrix algebra equations for transition probabilities - assuming that people's health can only deteriorate   95

Table 6: Example of a transition probability matrix: Quintile 1 Males moving from the 45-54 age group to the 55-64 age group   97

Figure 13: Age specific disability rates in the 1993 ABS survey and in DYNAMOD for 1986 and 1998   101

Figure 14: Proportion of disabled in the Australian population by health states, ABS survey and DYNAMOD, 1998   103

Figure 15: Age-specific fertility rates: simulated average for 1994 to 1998 and ABS actual figures for 1996   109

Table 7: Number of deaths by age, 1998 and 2018   117

Table 8: Number of disabled by age, 1998 and 2018   119

Figure 16: Proportion disabled in the population, Base case and Scenario, 1998 and 2018   119

Figure 17: Proportion disabled by health state, Base case and Scenario, 1998 and 2018   120

Figure 18: Expenditure on selected diseases* in 2000-01   121

Table 9 –Health expenditures* on the disabled by age, 1998 and 2018   122

Table 10: Logistic regressions, 45-54 year olds, variables influencing whether 'working',^ 1998 133

Figure 19: Distribution of the 45-54 and 65-70 populations by health state, ABS Survey and DYNAMOD, Base case, 1998   137

Figure 20: Per cent of 45-54 and 65-70 populations 'working' by health state,* ABS survey and DYNAMOD, Base case, 1998   138

Table 11: Persons* aged 65-70 years by health status, Base case and Scenario, 1998 and 2018 140

Table 12: Number of 65-70 year olds working more than 15 hours per week, Base case and Scenario, 1998 and 2018 141

Table 13: Mean weekly cash incomes of 45-54 year olds who worked more than 15 hours per week and whose main source of income was from wages and salaries, by health state (1998 dollars) 142

Table 14: Annual earnings* of 65 to 70 year olds, Base case and Scenario, 1998 and 2018 (1998 dollars) 143

Table 15: Assumptions made when estimating age pension expenditures on 65-70 year olds, Base case and Scenario, 1998 and 2018 145

Table 16: Potential savings on the age pension of 65 to 70 year olds if their employment patterns* were similar to that of 45 to 54 year olds in 1998, 1998 and 2018 (1998 dollars) 146

Table A1.1: Program structure – original version of DYNAMOD 177

Table A1.2: List of key DYNAMOD variables 181

Figure A4.2: Mortality rates, non-external causes (ie the disabled population), by age and sex, 1990-92 and 1995-97 198

Figure A4.3: Mortality rates, all causes by age and SEIFA quintiles, 1995-7 199

Figure A5.1: Disability rates by age and sex, 1993 and 1998 200

Figure A7.2.1: Proportion of Males by age group and disability level, 1998 210

Figure A7.2.2: Proportion of Females by age group and disability level, 1998 210

Figure A7.3.1: Proportion of population disabled (mild and severe), by equivalent income quintile, 1998 211

Table A7.4.1: Proportion of persons aged 15 years or more by health and labour force status, 1998 (per cent) 212

Table A7.4.2: Proportion of total population in private dwellings and institutions, 1998 (per cent) 213

Figure A7.5.2: Proportion of population with one, two …nine conditions, 1998 215

Table A9.1: Main reason as to why not looking for work, by age, 1998 217

x

Definitions

Age pension age	refers to the age, set by legislation, after which Australians may be eligible for government support through the age pension. During our study period the age pension age was 65 years for men and 60 years for women.
Core activities	Communication, mobility and self care (ABS 1999c, p.66)
Core activity restriction	Four levels based on whether 'needs help', 'has difficulty', or 'uses aids/equipment' with a core activity task. *Profound*: unable to do or always needs help. *Severe*: sometimes needs help. *Moderate*: needs no help but has difficulty. *Mild*: needs no help/has no difficulty, but uses aids/equipment (ABS 1999c, p.66).
Dependent	Children under 16 years of age, and full-time dependent students up to 25 years of age
Disability	A limitation, restriction or impairment, which has lasted, or is likely to last, for at least six months and restricts every day activities (ABS 1999c, pp.66-7)
Enhanced model	The DYNAMOD model as at August 2004, with elements of the Health_SES and Health state transition module incorporated.
Family	ABS (2003, Appendix 1) defines 'income unit' as adults and dependent children within a household whose income is shared. The concept is close to that of a family. In this thesis 'family' is generally used as a proxy for 'income unit'.
Long term health condition/illness	A long term health condition is a disease or disorder, including damage from accidents or injuries, which has lasted, or is likely to last, for six months or more (ABS 2000, p.3)
Equivalent family income (or wealth)	Gross annual family cash income (or wealth), 'needs-adjusted' to account for differences in family size.
The health states modelled	'No illness or disability': has neither long term health condition nor disability;
	'Long term illness': has long term health illness or condition but no disability;
	'Disabled_severe retriction': has disability and is profoundly, severely or moderately restricted in core activities;
	'Disabled_mild restriction': has disability and is either not restricted or mildly restricted in core activities.

Symbols (used in section 4.4)

$l^a_{x,y}$ number in able–bodied population aged x within SES quintile y

$l^d_{x,y}$ number in disabled population aged x within SES quintile y

$q^a_{x,y}$ mortality rates for the able–bodied population aged x within SES quintile y

$q^d_{x,y}$ mortality rates for the disabled population aged x within SES quintile y

$q_{x,y}$ mortality rates for the general population aged x within SES quintile y

$p_{x,y}$ prevalence of disability at age x within SES quintile y

$\theta_e(x_1 x_2, y)$ number of deaths due to external causes between ages x_1 and x_2 within SES quintile y

$\theta(x_1 x_2, y)$ total number of deaths between ages x_1 and x_2 in SES quintile y

$R_{x,y}$ number of recoveries from disability aged x within SES quintile y

$D_{x,y}$ number of people becoming disabled aged x within SES quintile y

$E_{x,y}$ initial number exposed to risk for the entire population at age x within SES quintile y

$r_{x,y}$ rate of decrement among the disabled due to recovery at age x, in SES quintile y

$d_{x,y}$ rate of decrement due to people becoming disabled at age x within SES quintile y

$\theta^a_{x,y}$ number of deaths in the able–bodied population at age x within SES quintile y

$\theta^d_{x,y}$ number of deaths in the disabled population aged x within SES quintile y

$\delta(x, y, i)$ percentage change in the total mortality rate in the ith year at age x within SES quintile y

NOTE: the above variables were also a function of sex and time. However, in the notation these variables were omitted for sake of simplicity of presentation.

Abbreviations

ABS	Australian Bureau of Statistics
AIHW	Australian Institute of Health and Welfare
Disability survey	Disability, Ageing and Carers surveys by the ABS
NHS	National Health Survey conducted by the ABS.
SES	Socioeconomic status

Chapter 1 Overview

This Chapter presents an overview of the research described in the thesis. Briefly, it concerns the further development of an existing dynamic microsimulation model of the Australian population to consider health and socioeconomic issues as they affect people's quality of life, their personal finances and government expenditures. The original and novel parts of the thesis are in Chapters 4, 5, 6, 7, 8, 9, 11 and 12. Most of the related research had appeared, or are to appear, in six refereed publications: Walker (2002), Walker (2004a, 2004b) and Walker and Becker (2005).

1.1   Introduction

1.1.1 Background

It is generally recognised that the dramatic gains in the health of Australians over the past century owed at least as much to social policies than to health policies. Glasson (2004) notes that it was social, economic and environmental conditions that have dictated the patterns of illness and disease in that period. Initially, improved water supplies and better housing and sanitation had the greatest impact on people's longevity. Later better hygiene, new medical technology, preventive medicine and people becoming more aware of their own health - through improved public education – further improved health and longevity. However, not all Australians benefited equally from these developments, with people of low socioeconomic status (SES) having worse health than those with higher SES (Chapter 2).

In recent years health inequalities became a much-researched subject, with a number of developed countries having already announced policies that aim to reduce inequalities in health – eg Acheson (1998) and King's Fund (1999) for the UK, and McCain and Mustard (1999 and 2002) for Canada.

Much of the research published in Australia and overseas concerns differences in mortality patterns across socioeconomic status (SES) at a particular point in time. The virtually universal finding is that people with low SES – usually the 'poor' – die younger than people with high SES – usually the 'rich' (World Health Organization, 2000; Glover et al, 1999). More recently research concerning the patterns of premature death by the socially disadvantaged has started to broaden out to consideration of the reasons why premature death is more common amongst the poor. Examples are the study of individuals' health and lifestyles as they impact on mortality rates (Marmot, 1998).

Authors of several recent publications expressed preference for a *life course* approach, partly because they saw health in later years of life as being the result of the accumulation of health related practices and events over time, and because health issues were seen to affect several facets of people's lives from birth to death (Davey Smith, 2002; Kuh and Ben-Shlomo (eds), 1997). Others found that socioeconomic status had implications for a wide range of outcomes over the life course, the impact on health being only one of these. For example, Tomison and Wise (1999) found that considerable benefits arose from the Perry project – which intervened at the preschool level in a low SES area of the United States - in terms of better health, less need for welfare services, less unemployment, and lower crime rates than in the control group some two decades after the intervention took place (section 2.7).

Many are of the view that the world is now entering a new era in medicine, health care and life expectancy. Reasons for this include the development of new therapies in the wake of the publishing - in 2000 - of the Human Genome sequence, and the rapid advances in the related area of proteomics.[1] For example, new medicines recently listed on Australia's Pharmaceutical Benefits Scheme now allow patients with previously fatal diseases to live a normal life. Because of the very high cost of such drugs, and the life and death decisions involved with their access, the adequacy of some well-tried and well-accepted existing policies are now being re-examined (Brown et al, 2002).

Also, new technologies are currently being researched to alleviate the impact of ageing related degenerative diseases, such as Alzheimer's and arthritis (Doherty, 2001).[2] Kirkwood (2001) notes that, although in the next few decades life expectancies are likely to increase well beyond current predictions, the focus in future is likely to be on improved quality of life as people age.

In such a new era a capacity to study the complex links between disease and mortality patterns over the life course, and to analyse the financial and equity effects of possible responses – as is done in this thesis - will be particularly important.

1.1.2   Aims of thesis

The aim of this thesis is to make a unique contribution to the general trend toward a life course approach in studies of health by socioeconomic status through development of a capacity to:

---

[1] Proteomics concerns proteins, the end products of genes.

2 Professor Doherty won the Nobel Prize for Medicine in 1996.

- analyse the complex links between disease and mortality patterns over the life course and across socioeconomic groups (to be achieved through the building of a Health_SES module);

- study the impact of health on people's functionality in terms of their ability to work or to live independently (to be achieved through the building of a Health State Transition module).

The two new modules are to be attached to an existing dynamic microsimulation model of the Australian population - the Health_SES module aiming to allow the health of the population to be analysed by SES groups, and the Health State Transition module to address the issue of how health affects people's functionality. A further aim is to validate the enhanced model.

Although the focus of the thesis is on model building, two topical and policy relevant applications have been included to illustrate the enhanced model's capabilities. These could be improved in future as the model is developed further – for example under the mid-2005 to mid-2008 Australian Research Council grant, which will see the model developed to the stage of a decision-making tool for use by policy analysts.

1.2   Reasons for choosing dynamic microsimulation

1.2.1   Background

The OECD (1996) has referred to microdata and microsimulation modelling as being among the few newer sophisticated techniques available to analysts in the health economics and population ageing fields.

Microsimulation, pioneered by Guy Orcutt in the US in the 1950s (Orcutt 1957; Orcutt et al 1961) is based on analysing the impact of social and economic policies by simulating the behaviour of and characteristics of individual decision-making units. Whereas in traditional studies the unit of analysis is a group of people with a common set of characteristics and behaviour patterns, in microsimulation the unit is the individual, with his or her rich set of personal characteristics.

Microdata (that is, information at the person level) is available through data collections - such as the Census - and relates to individuals as well as their families. Models can be constructed using such microdata. Because they deal with the individual, use of such models allows the impact of policy changes to be examined in far greater detail than is possible with more traditional approaches.

Dynamic microsimulation models follow individuals over the life course. Initially they were built for operative use in forecasting and for policy recommendations – Klevmarken (1997). Current applications include forecasting, policy recommendation and the explanation of social phenomena. Dynamic microsimulation models are the result of a synthesis of various elements, and usually include a population database - empirical or synthetic; a facility to project this database into the future; a representation of alternative government policies (most commonly tax-benefit systems); and a series of behavioural elements.

With regard to forecasting models, microsimulation and cell-based approaches are often two alternatives to making similar statements about future population characteristics (Van Imhoff and Post 1998). While population projections (by age and sex) are generally produced by the cell-based cohort-component method (eg ABS 1996c), for projections with the broad range of variables required in policy relevant life course studies microsimulation was found to be the most appropriate method – Spielaue (2002).

O'Donoghue (2001) describes recent research in dynamic microsimulation modelling in the UK, Canada, the USA, Australia, Sweden and Italy. The simpler and less computer 'hungry' *static* - ie 'snapshot'- versions of *microsimulation* models are now routinely used worldwide in policy analyses, especially in the tax and 'transfers' (ie social security) fields - see, for example, Orcutt et al (1986), Harding (1996), Nelissen (1996) and National Research Council (1991).

Adoption of large-scale dynamic microsimulation models has been slower. These are called 'dynamic' because in such models the life courses of individuals and their families are followed over time. Individual decisions are usually modelled based on historically observed patterns. Reasons for the slower 'take-up' of such models include their much longer development period (7 to 10 years) and hence development costs; their requirement for powerful computing equipment; and their complexity – making their use by non-specialists difficult. However, such models have the great advantage of bringing data together in a coherent fashion from many unrelated sources. The end result is that individuals (and their families) can be studied in considerable detail as they progress through the life course.

Recently dynamic microsimulation models have started to be used as sophisticated tools for policy-relevant analysis. Examples of the social, economic and health issues they have addressed to date are:

- the study of the impact of possible future changes to pension policies (Caldwell 1996; Frederiksen and Stolen 2003);

- simulation of the incomes and assets of older people and their ability to contribute towards home care costs in the UK (Hancock et al 2002);

- a study of how the UK and other European tax systems account for families (O'Donoghue and Sutherland 1999);

- an analysis of dental service use and expenditures in the US (Brown et al 1992, 1995);

- a study of which groups in Australia benefit more (or less) from government health expenditures over the life course (Harding et al 2002, also mentioned in section 2.5); and

- projections of the familial impact of AIDS on the elderly of Thailand (Wachter et al 2001).

Examples of existing dynamic microsimulation models are: DYNASIM and CORSIM for the United States; PENSIM and SAGE for the United Kingdom; DYNACAN and LifePaths for Canada; MOSART for Norway; and SESIM for Sweden. These models are described in section 2.6.

1.2.2   Reasons for choosing dynamic microsimulation

A key advantage of dynamic microsimulation compared with cell-based macro-models is that while cell-based models are limited to a few variables, microsimulation have many additional dimensions (eg individuals' risk exposures and their particular tax, insurance and social security profiles) - Spielaue (2002). Other advantages of microsimulation models are that distributional and other analyses can take account of many more variables *simultaneously*, and *interactions* between these variables can be modelled in considerably more complex ways than with traditional methods - Zaidi and Rake (2001. In this latter respect, Butler (1996) reported that allowing for consideration of more individual characteristics and for all possible combinations of these was likely to result in exponential increases in the number of cells in the data matrices that underpin traditional methods. In other words, while in macrosimulation models each additional variable produces an *exponential* increase in the size of the model, variables added to a microsimulation model have more of a *linear* effect on model size - provided that these variables are part of the initial micro-dataset (Walker 1997 and Department of Housing and Regional Development 1995).

A further advantage is that decision-making processes can be modelled at the level of the individual and/or their families and, when studying the impact of policy changes, the related changes in rules can be simulated as they apply to individuals (or families) in the real world. This applies to both static and dynamic microsimulation models.

As seen in section 1.2.1, a common application of microsimulation models is the study of the impact of possible future changes to pension policies (Caldwell 1996; Frederiksen and Stolen 2003). Also, a possible application that is of relevance to this thesis is the basing of the decision by one spouse to retire from the workforce on a range of factors such the health of each family member, the family's income and size, and the availability of carers.

The advantage of being able to model government policies by applying policy changes to individuals (or families) *directly* is that this mirrors the way public servants administer the policies in practice. This feature of microsimulation is particularly beneficial when considering a range of complex policies with simultaneous impact on families – hence the initial popularity of microsimulation techniques in the fields of tax and social security. Static microsimulation techniques have been applied to the health and aged care areas in: Caldwell et al (1993) and Wolf (2002) in the United States; Walker et al (2000) in Australia; and Health Canada (2001) in Canada.

Apart from their significant disadvantages (section 1.2.1), dynamic microsimulation models have many advantages over their static counterparts, such as their ability to project into the future; to follow individuals and their families over the life course; and to account for the accumulation of certain variables, such as savings and wealth at the family level - Walker (1997 and 1998). After conducting a review of existing models, Zaidi and Rake (2001) concluded that:

> "the prospect of building a dynamic microsimulation model may seem … daunting. However … there is now a critical mass of international expertise in this area. Many models are now in their second, third or even later generations. Each new model reflects a considerable amount of learning that followed from building the previous model. The challenge … in developing a new microsimulation model … is to capitalise on this expertise "

As noted in section 1.1.2, the work reported in this thesis should be seen in the light of this continuum – with the next generation of DYNAMOD already being developed.

Overall, although more time consuming and costly than other methods (section 1.2.1), dynamic microsimulation was chosen as the preferred modelling technique for this thesis due to the considerable advantages of using such techniques in complex studies covering the life course.

1.3 New modules as part of an existing model versus a stand-alone model

For this thesis there was a choice of building two stand-alone health models, specially built to track individuals' health status for particular applications, or the grafting of the same health status processes onto an existing, more comprehensive model. The key advantage of the former option would have been its relative simplicity – especially if tracking was limited to particular cohorts, as in Harding et al (2002)[3] and Wolf (2002). However, using the 'stand alone' method, the modelling of health in a comprehensive way in a socioeconomic context would have been well beyond the scope of a single

---

[3] See section 2.5 for a description of an application of that Australian model to the health field.

PhD project - unless it was so simplistic that its application to policy relevant issues became purely of academic interest. Because of this, the 'grafting of modules onto an existing model' option was chosen.

A key advantage of this option is that it allows the incorporation of a broader range of real life events and decisions that occur during the life courses of individuals and their families. By choosing an existing model that is based on high quality data and methods, and has been validated by earlier researchers (section 1.4), we can ensure that work on this thesis starts from a strong initial base.

1.4 The dynamic microsimulation model chosen

Because there is only one full population dynamic microsimulation model for Australia – DYNAMOD – it was the model chosen for purposes of this thesis. Its development evolved over a period of some ten years, so using it as part of this thesis was expected to considerably enhance the type of policy relevant applications that could be studied (section 1.6). The model – which has been extensively documented[4] - is able to project the entire Australian population to 2050. Appendix A1 describes the original version of DYNAMOD, including its Wealth module – that is, the model that existed before addition of the Health_SES and Health State Transition modules.

Briefly, the model is based on a 1 per cent representative sample of the population (150,000 persons) extracted by the Australian Bureau of Statistics (ABS) from its 1986 Census. Its original version, which was developed at the National Centre for Social and Economic Modelling, University of Canberra, it simulates future events occurring in the

---

[4] Stage 1 of the original model is documented in Antcliff (1993) and Antcliff et al (1996). King et al (1999b) provide an overview of stage 2 of DYNAMOD's development, with details and calibration in Abello et al (2002), Bækgaard (2002 a and b), King et al (2002), Walker (2000a), King et al (1999a) and Robinson and Bækgaard (2002). Stage 3 is described in Kelly (2002; 2003).

lives of persons in its base population - such as births, deaths, immigration, emigration, couple formation, education, employment, earned income, taxes, government transfers, superannuation, savings and the accumulation of wealth. Disability – defined as a limitation, restriction or impairment, which has lasted, or is likely to last, for at least six months and restricts every day activities (ABS 1999c)[5] - was modelled in the original version. However, in that version it played a relatively minor role as it was only linked to the rest of the model through the mortality and the education modules.

While some modules – such as death and fertility – are based on survival functions (which determine duration times), others – such as education and employment - are based on transition probabilities. For these latter the model uses the Monte Carlo method to allocate various event states to the individuals in its population base. It usually drawing a random number, z, from a uniform distribution over the interval [0, 1], usually comparing it with an estimated probability. This introduces randomness in the model results as different runs of the model, with identical parameters but using different random number seeds, will produce different outputs.

The order in which the modules for the various events are executed in the main simulation loop – monthly for most and yearly for some events – is in line with the typical progression of these in real life (Antcliff et al 1995, p. 19). In the original model this order was programmed as: first, earnings (if July), then emigration, death, disability, education (if January), leaving home (if January), labour force status, births, immigration, couple formation and, finally, couple dissolution – see King et al (1999b). Wealth, taxation and social security benefits (ie income from government), which were added to a later version of the model, are processed after earnings.

---

[5] A more detailed definition of 'disability' is in section 3.2.

The state-of-the-art techniques adopted in the early years of DYNAMOD's development are still chosen for new models currently being developed (section 2.6). Also, as seen above, the model is based on good quality – though mainly cross-sectional – data, and it has been validated against published official statistics (section 9.1). Details of the many variables available in DYNAMOD are in Table A1.2, Appendix A1. The author of this thesis gained familiarity with DYNAMOD when involved with the development of its immigration module (Walker 2000a and King et al 2002).

A basic philosophy when building both the original and this thesis version of DYNAMOD was to keep the model as close as possible to high quality 'real' – rather than 'synthetic' – data.[6] This method was, and is still preferred by builders of dynamic microsimulation models (section 2.6). Adoption of such a philosophy is seen as enhancing the model's credibility and thus its use by decision makers (section 2.6; Chapter 8). In this context, the ABS's 1 per cent Census sample is the most comprehensive data available to Australian researchers at the individual (ie unit record) level. As with most of its unit record files, the ABS has ensured that its 1986 Census sample is representative of Australia's full population.

DYNAMOD's extensive code – comprised of over 60 modules with complex inter-connections and close to 100 variables - is described in Appendix A1. The code is written in the C programming language, and was initially run on a UNIX system. The dramatic increases over the past decade in the speed and memory size of PCs resulted in a PC version of the model now being available - with each simulation generally taking 2 to 3 hours to run. It is this PC version that was modified and used in the thesis.

---

[6] Data drawn from statistical collections, such as the Census in DYNAMOD, is considered 'real' data. while base population data generated by the model itself – such as the full life histories of individuals in different birth cohorts in LifePaths – is defined as 'synthetic' data (eg) – see section 2.6.

With each run the model outputs the characteristics of each person, year-by-year, over the simulation period (or month-by-months for some variables), together with their family linkages. From these cross-sectional output files life histories can be created for each person simulated. Some SAS programs have been developed to analyse this massive output, mainly in a cross sectional framework – that is on year-by-year basis. These SAS programs take about an hour to run. It would be a considerable programming effort to develop a similar facility for analysing DYNAMOD's output in a longitudinal framework – for example to study health expenditures over the lifetime of individuals (rather than at one point in time only). For this reason, analyses covering the life course have not been conducted for this thesis.

In recent years C has been superseded by C++. As a result, the C language is no longer taught at most Universities. The model's C code is currently compiled by the latest available C++ complier. While the C++ compiler is able to handle programs written in C, it is not able to handle a program with mixed C and C++ code. Because of this the alterations and additions to the DYNAMOD code carried out for this thesis were written in the C language.

1.5   Steps involved in adding new modules to DYNAMOD

This section first presents the key elements that make up the enhanced version of DYNAMOD. Section 1.4 described the order in which events are processed in the original model. Processing of the new Health_SES and Health State Transition modules was inserted after the 'Wealth, taxation and social security benefits' module.[7]

---

[7] An explanation is provided in Section 4.1 as to why SES is computed *before* health states are considered.

Next, the section briefly describes the main tasks involved in adding the new

Health_SES and Health State Transition modules to the main model. When relevant,

the challenges encountered - and the way they had been overcome - are discussed in the

Chapters (or sections) indicated in brackets next to the step being considered. Finally,

the section provides an insight into the considerable programming effort that was

carried out for purposes of this thesis.

1.5.1 *Key elements of the enhanced model*

Figure 1 provides a schematic representation of the various elements that make up the

enhanced version of DYNAMOD.

Briefly, three main datasets are required as inputs to the model: Block 1 for data on the

individuals and their families whose life courses are to be simulated, the Base data in

the base year, 1986;[8] Block 2 for the input data needed for the new Health_SES and

Health State Transitions modules; and Block 3 for the remaining input data needed by

the original version of DYNAMOD (Appendix A1).

---

[8] With all the variables needed in the simulation period which are not available from
Census 1986 imputed.

Figure 1: **Elements of the enhanced version of DYNAMOD**

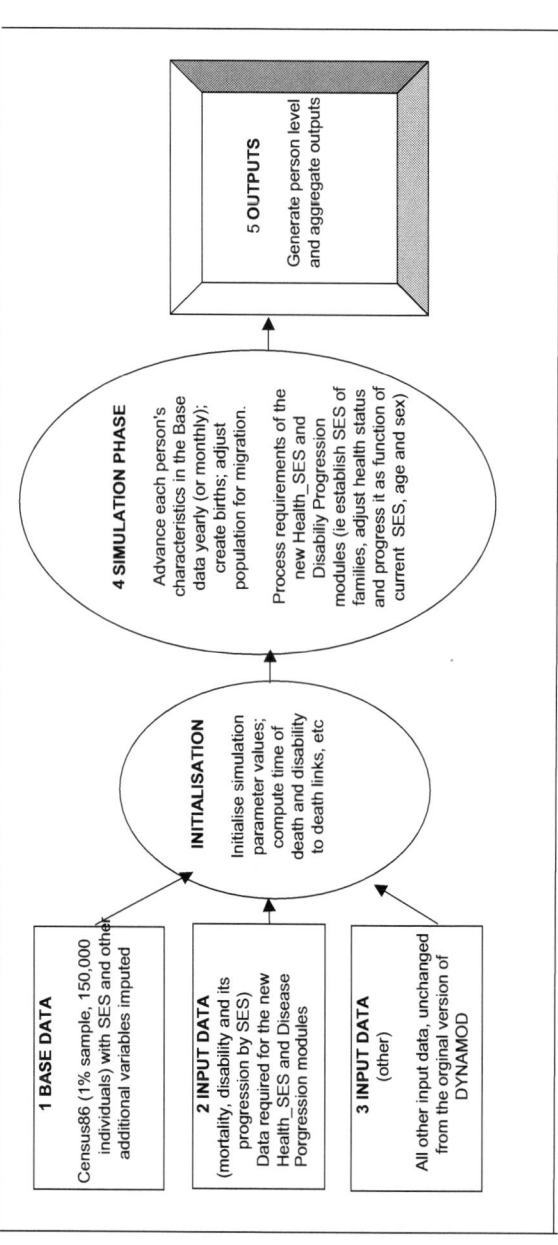

After 'initialising' the data in Block 1 with all the person-level characteristics for 1986, the simulation phase can commence (Block 4). During this phase each member of the Base population is advanced from one year to the next. Block 4 is thus the 'heart' of the model. During this phase the events occurring the lives of people are simulated over the specified time period – in this thesis from 1986 to 2018.

The final phase, Block 5, is one in which person-level and aggregate output statistics are computed and stored. They can then be used for further analyses – usually carried out outside DYNAMOD using the SAS programming language.

1.5.2 *The main steps*

The main steps involved in adding the two new modules to DYNAMOD are:

- reviewing the extensive literature on health inequalities and on choices for model building (Chapter 2);

- familiarisation with the techniques of dynamic microsimulation modelling; studying the structure, variables, and capabilities of the original version of DYNAMOD (Appendix A1); detailed study of the DYNAMOD code – which first required the learning of the C programming language (section 1.5.3);

- listing the variables required for constructing the new modules, separately identifying which of these could be constructed from the variables already in the model and which will need to be input into DYNAMOD (or imputed onto that model's base population) - section 4.3, and Chapters 6 and 8;

- establishing the linkages between variables that the enhanced model is to account for - eg health status is to account for age, sex and socioeconomic status (Chapters 4, 6; Appendix A1);

- searching for data sources that cover the new variables as well as the related desired linkages (Chapter 3; section 8.1);

- imputing the new variables onto individuals in DYNAMOD's Base dataset (section 7.1);

- preparing the new data in the required format to be input into DYNAMOD's initialisation and simulation phases - eg on health status and on its progression (Chapter 6; sections 8.2 and 8.4.1);

- reading the new input data needed for the simulation phase of DYNAMOD, initialising it, programming the required linkages between the new variables and the ones already in DYNAMOD, and programming in the year-by-year progression of these variables throughout the model's simulation period (sections 1.4, 1.5.3; Chapters 7, 11, 12; Appendix A1);

- programming in the aggregations required for outputting the required results, and the storing of such DYNAMOD results for further analyses (sections 1.4, 1.5.1).

1.5.3   The programming effort

The programming effort involved with the grafting of the two new modules onto the existing model, took up over half of the total time spent on this thesis. As mentioned in section 1.4, the programming languages used were C (with C++ compiler) for the modules added to the original version of DYNAMOD, and SAS for the analysis of ABS survey data and the voluminous DYNAMOD outputs. While the author was familiar with the SAS language, she needed to learn the C and C++ programming languages before a detailed study of the DYNAMOD code could be undertaken. The texts used to do this were Horton (1998), Stroustrup (1992), Kernigan and Ritchie (1988), and Kelley and Pohl (1990).

Once the C and C++ languages were sufficiently understood and the structure of the DYNAMOD code had been examined in detail, the two new modules were programmed into the main model as follows.

Each time the month of July is reached during the simulation period, a new sub-program program:

- reads in the required externally specified and model generated data files;

- computes family level socioeconomic status indicators for each person in that year's DYNAMOD population; sorts these from lowest to highest SES and divides them into five parts (quintiles), each comprising 20% of the population;

- determines, for each person, whether a transition in health state will take place that year, given the person's current health state, age, sex and socioeconomic status;

- estimates the probability of working , for the application in Chapter 12, and allocates work status to the relevant sub-population; and

- computes aggregate statistics - such as number of persons by health state, by age and SES that year, or total population that year – and arranges for these to be added to DYNAMOD's standard output files.

In addition, numerous links had to programmed between the above sub-program and the code of the original model. The original code comprises over 40 programs, a selection of which is listed in Table A1.1 (Appendix A1). Those parts of the original code that were modified for this thesis have been **bolded** in that Table. The C code for the sub-program written specifically for purposes of this thesis is available to examiners on request.

1.6 Questions the enhanced model may address

Use of the enhanced model allows researchers:

- to study the implications for quality of life and for health expenditures of possible improvements in public health (in aggregate or separately for various age, sex or SES groups) – see Chapter 11;

- to assess the implication of a person's health and family situation on his/her ability to remain in the labour force (Chapter 12);

- to consider the distributional impact of government spending on health and social security *simultaneously*;

  o together with the impact of such spending on families in different socioeconomic groups;

- to assess levels of dependency at older ages, based on the interaction of a person's health status with changes in his/her economic or family circumstances; and

- to study people's capacity for self-funding their own retirement under different assumption regarding the level of public health in Australia.

With further development of the model - section 13.2 - additional policy relevant questions could be added to the above list.

1.7   Outline of thesis

The thesis is structured in three parts, with an overview - *Chapter 1*- preceding these. The overview sets out the reasons why the topics covered in the thesis are important; specifies the aims of the thesis; explains why the technique of dynamic microsimulation was chosen and why the grafting of new modules to an existing model was preferred to two new 'stand alone' models. It concludes with a list topical issues that could be studied on completion of the planned modelling effort, followed by an outline of the thesis.

Part 1 concerns the development of the Health_SES and Health State Transition modules, including:

- what is currently known from the literature (Chapter 2);

- the data used (Chapter 3 and section 8.1);

- the methodologies adopted for the Health_SES module (Chapter 4), including the complex set of equations that link disability to mortality by SES (section 4.4);

- a regression analysis of the relative importance of the various determinants of income (section 4.3);

- the methodologies adopted for the Health State Transition module (section 8.3), including a novel method for estimating health transition probabilities from cross sectional data (in the absence of longitudinal data);

- quantitative analyses that aim to establish whether the geographic area-based SES indicators or the individual level income-based indicators are preferable for purposes of this thesis (Chapter 5);

- description of how the mortality and disability input datasets required by the new modules were prepared (Chapter 6, sections 8.2 and 8.4.1);

- documentation of how health states and socioeconomic status were modelled within the simulation phase of DYNAMOD (Chapters 7 and 8);

- validation of the enhanced model (Chapter 9);

- limitations of the enhanced model – including the need for better alignment methodologies (Chapter 10).

Part 2 provides two illustrative applications of the enhanced model, one estimating the personal and social implications of a narrowing of health inequalities in Australia (Chapter 11), and the other studying the impact of health on older person's ability to remain in the labour force (Chapter 12). The material in the first twelve Chapters is supported by evidence and methodological details presented in eleven Appendices.

Part 3 presents the overall conclusions of the thesis and discusses possible future extensions and improvements to the model (Chapter 13).

PART 1: DEVELOPMENT OF THE HEALTH_SES AND HEALTH STATE TRANSITION MODULES

23

Chapter 2   Relevant findings from the literature

In this Chapter we report on findings from the literature that could be relevant either to the research carried out for this thesis, or for the possible future developments mentioned in Chapter 13. The studies quoted have either appeared in reputable Journals, or in publications by well respected government or international organisations. They are thus generally considered to be of high quality.

2.1 Mortality based studies of the health-SES links

Numerous studies worldwide have found that people with lower socioeconomic status die younger than do people with higher socioeconomic status - World Health Organisation (2000), Glover et al (1999), Marmot (1998). This pattern is evident in developed as well as in developing countries, indicating that it is relative rather than absolute differences that matter – Saunders (1996). For Australia, a recent study estimated that

Many Australian studies used mortality as the indicator of health status and the geographic area of the last residence prior to death as a proxy for socioeconomic status (Turrel and Mathers 2001; Dunn et al, 2002; Vinson 1999; Gregory and Hunter 1995).[9] A recent study of this kind estimated that, in 1998-2000, life expectancy at birth was 79.2 years for Australian men born in the least disadvantage areas compared with 75.3 years for those born in the most disadvantaged areas. For corresponding figures for females were 83.6 and 81.6 years respectively (Draper et al, 2004).

---

[9] In mortality studies occupation – at the level of the individual, usually grouped as blue/white collar - is also a widely used measure of SES (see for example Draper et al 2004 and AIHW 2005).

Use of geographic area of residence as an SES indicator is facilitated by the Australian

Bureau of Statistics computing, within its Censuses, Socioeconomic Indexes for Areas

(SEIFA) at the Census Collector District level (ABS 1998c and 1991b). Details on

SEIFA indexes are in Appendix A3.

Figure 2 – reproduced from a report by the Australian Institute of Health and Welfare,

Mathers et al (1999) - illustrates the typical findings of studies of this kind. It shows that

in the mid-1990s Australian men in the most disadvantaged SES quintile (Q5) had an

18% chance of dying between ages 25 and 65, compared with 12% for men in the least

disadvantaged quintile (Q1). For women, although the probability of dying was

consistently lower, the range still varied significantly (from 7 to 10 per cent).

Figure 2:   **Probability of Australians aged 25–65 years dying, by sex and quintile of
socioeconomic disadvantage, 1995–97**

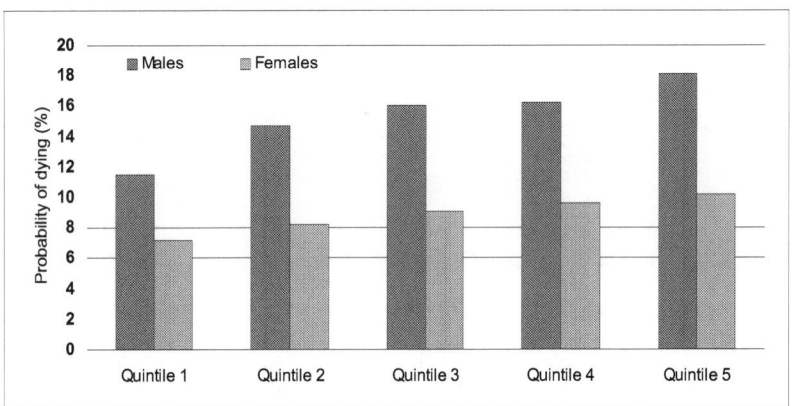

Note: The quintiles are by social and economic disadvantage of area of residence. Quintile 1 is
the least disadvantaged, and quintile 5 the most disadvantaged.
Source: Mathers, Vos and Stevenson (1999, p. 39).

The statistical associations illustrated in Figure 2 should not be seen simply as a gap in

death rates between those living in the most and least disadvantaged geographical areas, but rather as a gradient – or change in the same direction – across all socioeconomic groups.

There is evidence to suggest that policy interventions aimed at reducing mortality rates are more likely to be adopted by higher SES people than by others. For example Hayen et al (2002), who examined avoidable mortality over the 1980-2000 period, found that the uptake of primary interventions – eg smoking cessation, improved diet, increased physical activity – had a significantly greater impact on avoidable mortality amongst the least disadvantaged 20% of the population than in the rest of the population. A recent longitudinal UK study of mortality and health found that wealth was an important determinant of mortality and the evolution of health (Attanasio and Emmerson 2003).

The main implications of the above findings for this thesis are that:

- mortality rates and the SEIFA should be amongst the variables considered in this thesis (because mortality is an often used proxy for health status in the literature, and the SEIFA index an often used proxy for socioeconomic status);

- if possible, wealth should be included in the indicator of SES used, and

- the response to policy interventions which aim to reduce health inequalities is a complex one – placing full consideration of such interventions beyond the scope of this thesis.

2.2 Intergenerational effects

The literature suggests that the SES effects on health – apart from being evident at every stage of the life course - are 'transmitted' across generations. For example, an Australian study found that:

"parents who grew up in a socially disadvantaged situation during their own childhood have lower early age cognitive abilities, suggesting a potentially important cross-generational link that may well spill over to affect the subsequent economic fortunes of children of disadvantaged individuals." - Gregg and Machin (2000, p. 11).

This issue is of considerable concern to the governments in Australia, with policies having been introduced with an aim to break the 'cycle of inter-generational welfare dependency' - Newman (1999, p. 3).

Since dynamic microsimulation models track the life courses of individuals and their families, they are one of the few analytical tools able to account for intergenerational effects. While the modelling of such effects was beyond the scope of this thesis, such an exercise could in future be undertaken as an extension of this project (Chapter 13).

2.3 Labour market effects

The labour market effects of poor health are an important topic for this thesis. For the UK, Bartley and Owen (1996) found that limiting longstanding illness was strongly associated with economic inactivity, rather than with unemployment. They defined 'inactive' persons as being those neither in employment nor seeking work, and found that the 'economically inactive' were mostly the permanently sick, and the early retired. These authors also found that the tighter the labour market, the healthier a British man had to be to get a job, and that those in sufficiently poor health to affect their short term risk of mortality tended to join the ranks of the "permanently sick", rather than register as "unemployed and actively seeking work".

For Australia, Schofield (1996) found that lack of employment was associated with poorer than average health, and working many hours was associated with an increase in risk factors that could lead to health problems in the longer term.

Overall, the literature suggests that – in most developed countries - the seriously ill are unlikely to be in the labour force. As a consequence, those employed tend to have better than average health. The literature also suggests that those with jobs requiring long working hours may in the long run have worse than average health.

The links between health and employment status are the subject of the applications presented in Chapter 12.

2.4 Causality

As seen in section 2.3, the relationship between health and employment does not always operate in the same direction, with employment being associated with better health in some cases, but with worse health in others.

This raises the issue of causality, not only with respect to the health-employment relationships, but also the health-SES linkages. The question is whether low SES causes poor health, or poor health causes low earning capacity, and thus low socioeconomic status. While with cross-sectional data researchers are only able to identify statistical associations between these variables, with longitudinal data it is possible to identify the direction of causation. This is because in longitudinal data researchers are able to establish whether low income preceded poor health, or poor health preceded low income. This was recognised by the Forum on Research Study Design (1999), which noted that the biggest benefit of longitudinal studies was their ability to establish cause-and-effect relationships.

For the United States, a longitudinal study by Lynch et al (1997) found that, after abstracting from other factors, it was low income that caused poor health. These authors concluded that sustained economic hardship led to poorer physical, psychological and cognitive functioning, as well as ill health. They found little evidence of reverse causation — that is, that episodes of illness might have caused subsequent economic hardship. This is similar to the findings of the Marmot et al. (1991) study of British civil servants that:

"health-related downward mobility has been shown not to account for national social-class mortality differences" (p. 1392).

For Australians aged 15–24, a longitudinal study by Graetz (1993, p. 14) has shown that while unemployment (and thus low income) had adverse effects on health and wellbeing, health deterioration did not generally lead to unemployment.

However, there will be cases where severe illness will result in people withdrawing from the labour force and thus no longer earning income. This latter direction of causation is implied in a summary of the international literature by Bradbury et al (2001) who reported that a correlation existed between severe disability and low labour force participation, low employment rates and low income.

Overall, the longitudinal data based literature for developed countries suggests that in most cases it is low income that causes poor health (although there will be 'reverse causation' in a few instances). The finding that, in general, low income that causes poor health is made use of in the thesis when modelling the health_SES link (Chapter 4). The existence of the few instances of 'reverse causation' means that the model will over-estimate the impacts of income changes.

Regarding the impact of income inequality – as opposed to income per se - a recent review by Lynch et al (2004) found little support in developed countries for a direct effect of income inequality on health. These authors nevertheless concluded that reducing income inequality by raising the incomes of the poor improved their health, was likely to lead to narrower health inequalities and to improved population health.

This finding is made use of in the Chapter 11 application presented in the thesis (section 11.1).

2.5   Life course approach

Recent publications on the health-SES linkages have advocated the adoption of a life course approach. For example, Kuh and Ben-Shlomo (1997) mention UK studies which show that the risk of cardiovascular disease, diabetes and chronic bronchitis is higher among those born or brought up in poor childhood circumstances, or experienced poor growth in infancy. They note that such research suggests that environmental factors had programmed particular body systems during critical periods of growth - in utero and in infancy - with long term consequences for adult chronic disease. They also note that in the past forty years adult chronic disease has been the main public health issue in developed countries - with research focusing on adult risk factors (eg smoking, diet, exercise).

For Australia, Turrell et al (1999) found that socioeconomic differences in health were evident at every stage of the life course — from birth to infancy, childhood, adolescence and adulthood. They also found that 'premature death' of the socially disadvantaged tended to be associated with earlier onset of diseases than for the population generally.

Because dynamic microsimulation models simulate key events in the lives of individuals and their families (Chapter 1), they are particularly well suited to analyses covering the life course. One example of a cohort-based dynamic microsimulation model in the health area is described in Harding et al (2002). This research concerns the lifetime distributional impact of Australia's health expenditures funded by government. It answers questions such as: which groups in society benefit more (or less) from health-related government 'subsidies' when such expenditures are considered over the life courses of the cohorts studied. It thus takes into account the fact that for most people health needs are much greater early and late in life than during their working lives. This model was not chosen for use in this thesis because first because it does not represent the full Australian population since it is based on a pseudo-cohort of 4000 persons simulated from birth to death. Second, members of the pseudo-cohort live all of their lives in a steady-state world (Australia in 1986) and third, because it has a more limited set of variables than DYNAMOD (eg wealth accumulation is not modelled). Fourth, it lacks some of DYNAMOD's complex interactions between variables that are important for this thesis. In particular differential mortality is only modelled from age 45 onwards (as a function of education, age and sex), and is not linked to disability – a feature which does not allow assessment of life years saved as the health of the population improves.

2.6 Other countries' dynamic microsimulation models

Dynamic microsimulation models are now routinely used throughout the developed world, and there is an increasing demand for them in policy analyses (section 1.2.2). In the last few decades recognition of the importance of studying the 'life course' (section 2.5) was followed by integration of the structural and dynamic approaches to the life course paradigm. The result has been the combination of several major streams of research connecting social change, social structure and individual action (Giele and Elder 1998), leading to highly complex models able to analyse most of the important life-course factors simultaneously.

The types of microsimulation models developed to date and their characteristics are as follows (Spielaue 2002):

- cohort models, which age a single cohort over the entire lifetime. These typically investigate lifetime income and interpersonal distributions (eg Harding et al 2002);

- full population models. While these are considerably less restrictive in their applications than cohort models, they are usually far more complex and demanding with regard to data;

- models assuming 'steady-state' patterns – ie that base year probabilities will remain unchanged over time - versus models producing forecasts that reflect the expected future world;

- 'open' population models (in which spouses are found either in that country's population or are imported) versus 'closed' population models (in which spouses can only be found in that country's population). Whether an 'open' or a 'closed' population approach is chosen will strongly depend on how immigration is planned to be modelled.

As a first step in building a new dynamic microsimulation model for the UK – SAGE - Zaidi and Rake (2001) reviewed a selection of such models built since the 1970s. Details on models for countries other than Australia are as follows:[10]

- DYNASIM: the pioneering dynamic microsimulation model for the United States (1970s, University of Michigan and Social Security Adminiatration). It was re-developed as DYNASIM2 (1990s). The model accounts for most of the life events simulated in the original version of DYNAMOD.

- CORSIM, the first PC-based dynamic microsimulation model for the United States (late 1980s, Cornell University); now running in its fourth generation

---

[10] References are in brackets when not based on the Zaidi and Rake (2001) review.

32

version (Strategic Forecasting, a New York based policy research firm); has been instrumental in assisting the Social Security Administration in its Social Security Reform Analysis.

- PENSIM, a dynamic microsimulation model for the United Kingdom (Department of Social Security) to project the incomes of future pensioners. Further development is currently underway for the second version (adding disability status, retirement decisions, institutionalization, with possible use of aggregate macroeconomic trends to align the forecasts generated by the model).

- MOSART, the dynamic microsimulation model for Norway (late 1980s, Statistics Norway), built to study options for the financing of future public expenditures. Original version simulated too few events to be of general use; now in its third version. Disability is only accounted for once people qualify for a disability pension.

- SESIM, the dynamic microsimulation model of the Swedish population, which is similar to DYNAMOD. However, it also accounts for non-cash benefits (such as aged care, health care, medications) and allows for behavioural adjustment in its labour force module. Disability is only accounted for once people qualify for a disability pension - Fredriksen and Stolen (2003); Pettersson and Pettersson, (2003).

- LifePaths, the dynamic microsimulation model of Statistics Canada (developed over a decade; the only one of the models listed here with a synthetic base population and use of continuous time; generates full life history of individuals of various overlapping birth cohorts).

- DESTINIE, a dynamic microsimulation model for France (late 1990s), producing private sector pension projections; retrospective simulation of career paths; operational model much used for policy analysis; possible future extension to the public sector.

- DYNACAN, a longitudinal dynamic microsimualtion model for Canada (1990s, currently with Social Development and Communication Ministry). Iinitially a modified version of CORSIM. The Canadian government uses the model to project and assess the distributive impacts of changes to the Canada Pension Plan (Morrison 1999).

- SAGE, a dynamic microsimulation model currently being developed in the United Kingdom to study the impact of different social policy options on the future demand for pensions, health and personal social services, and long-term care (Evandrou et al, 2001).

The specifications of several of these models are similar to those adopted in DYNAMOD. For example most are based on high quality statistical collections - rather than on synthetically generated data; account for a similar set of life course variables; and in general model the relationships between these variables using logistic regressions based on historical data - rather than on mathematical functions fitted to such data. The fact that such characteristics are still chosen for new models currently being developed – Zaidi and Rake (2001) - increases the credibility of earlier models, such as DYNAMOD.

Another common characteristic of these models is that they are either developed for, or mainly used by, government organisations. Due to their complexity, it takes about a decade to develop dynamic microsimulation models to a stage suitable for policy analysis. For example, the new SAGE model, work on which commenced in late 1999, has not as yet been used to simulate a policy application.

The key reason why governments have persevered with funding the development and maintenance of such models, and that more are currently being built, is that there are applications where there are virtually no alternatives to microsimulation. Caldwell and Morrison (2000) give the following examples:

- projections of winners and losers of alternative policies (period specific or lifetime basis);

- studies that are *simultaneously* focussed on families and individuals;

- micro-level operation of the social security programs within the tax/transfer system;

- study of the choice to work or retire at particular life course or period junctures;

- study of the decisions to save;

- cross-subsidies across population groups or cohorts;

- feedback effects of government programs on population demographics;

- longer-term consequences of social trends in marriage, divorce and fertility.

Other areas in which there are virtually no alternatives to dynamic microsimulation include: studies of how wealth at the family level is accumulated over the life course; the availability of spouses/children as carer for the frail aged; the intergenerational transfer of wealth; and heredity transmission of specific health risks.

2.7 Discussion

Despite decades of intensive research worldwide, the reasons for the observed health-SES patterns, and for their consistency across countries, are still not well understood. The literature indicates that factors such as genetics, quality of health services and health risk factors (diet, smoking, blood pressure, physical activity, obesity, social support) can explain only part of the differences observed in health status or mortality rates. The remainder is thought by some to arise from the additional stress that the most disadvantaged experience due to their social environment, the lesser 'control' they have over their lives and the social and economic implications of low incomes - Marmot (1998).

Incomplete understanding of the reasons for the health-SES links, however, did not discourage social experimentation, especially interventions in the early years of children's lives – see for example Walker (2001a). Of particular importance is that, over the longer term, considerable savings were found to eventuate from such experimental projects. Tomison and Wise (1999) note in relation to the US Perry Preschool project that, as adults the Perry graduates showed better health as well as better social competence (measured across a series of indices relating to criminality, use of welfare services, family structure and career success) than the control group. These authors also reported on a cost-benefit analysis which showed that, by the time the Perry graduates reached age 27, for every US$1 spent on the Perry program, there was a subsequent saving of over US$7 dollars in terms of lower costs of health, welfare, crime fighting and the jail system.

The above suggests that the modelling of the health-SES-link in a life course context – as is done in this thesis - is highly policy relevant.

Chapter 3   Choice of Data Sources

This Chapter examines the data sources that could have been used when developing the new Health-SES and Health State Transition modules. The Chapter also indicates which of these sources were chosen and why.

3.1 Data requirements

Because dynamic microsimulation models track individuals over the life course, the data sources used to build such models should ideally be longitudinal in nature. At the Forum on Research Study Design (1999) it was noted that the biggest benefits of longitudinal studies were their ability to establish cause-and-effect relationships (particularly lifetime relationships), to identify emerging issues and to indicate transitions (for example, in and out of disease states). At that Forum it was also noted that, unlike many other developed countries, Australia had little data available through longitudinal surveys. For this reason, we mainly considered cross sectional data for the building of the Health-SES and Health State Transition modules.

Also, it was important that the unit record datasets chosen for developing the new modules were sufficiently large to allow disaggregation by a number of variables – such as age, sex, socioeconomic status, health status and employment status.

3.2   The data sources considered

The data needed to build the new modules fall into three categories:

    (a) imputation of SES (and other less important variables) to the base data;

(b) transformation of the age/sex disaggregation of the original model's input
datasets on mortality and on disability into ones by age, sex *and SES*; and

(c) preparation of a new input dataset on transition probabilities - associated with
progression to the various stages of disability by severity.

The data sources considered were: mortality statistics from the Australian Institute of
Health and Welfare (AIHW); causes of deaths published by the Australian Bureau of
Statistics (ABS); the Australian Longitudinal Study on Ageing; and the national health
and disability surveys by the ABS (Appendix A2).

The ABS's large nationwide unit record surveys - seemed particularly suitable for this
thesis. These were its then latest 1995 National Health Survey (NHS) – a household
survey - and the1993 and 1998 Disability surveys – which includes both households and
institutions. Their suitability was further investigated, with findings reported in section
3.3.

Disability is a particularly useful variable for this thesis because, on the one hand, it can
be linked to diseases through the 'main disabling condition' variable in the 1998
Disability survey (ABS 1999a) and, on the other, to a person's functionality. The survey
also contains comprehensive information on income – although, as with all income
collections, the data on the incomes of people aged 65 or more years is less accurate –
and varies less by SES – than those of the working population. A likely explanation of
these small differences is that 70% of people in that age group have sufficiently low
cash incomes to receive the age pension (Harding et al 2004). Thus the majority in that
age group will have low income-based socioeconomic status. Although older people are
the ones most likely to have accumulated wealth (Harding et al 2004), in common with
the NHSs, the Disability survey contains no data on wealth.

In line with proposals by the World Health Organisation (Appendix A2, section A2.3), the ABS's 1998 survey defines disability as a limitation, restriction or impairment which has lasted - or is likely to last - for at least six months and restricts every day 'core activities'. These core activities are grouped under the headings of communication, mobility and self care (ABS 1999b, pp.66-7). Definitions of core activities and other disability related variables are in section A2.3. Data availability on health states and on how disability accounts for the severity of a person's functional restrictions are discussed in section 8.1.

Although the recent HILDA (Household, Income and Labour Dynamics) survey – conducted by the Melbourne Institute of Applied Economic and Social Research at the University of Melbourne - is longitudinal and has wealth information, it was not considered because (i) its wave 2 data only became available after the simulations for this thesis had been completed; and (ii) it has very limited information on health.

The other longitudinal data source, the Australian Longitudinal Study on Ageing, was considered and subjected to further examination. It is a potentially useful data source since it brings together information on the health, social and economic circumstances of older Australians. After further examination, however, it was not chosen for use in this thesis because of its small sample size (2,087 participants in wave 1) and because all those in the study lived in the Adelaide metropolitan area. The survey's small size meant that disaggregation by all the variables of interest to this thesis would not have been possible. Also, the full sample having been drawn from Adelaide meant that the data could not be considered to be representative of all Australians.

The data sources selected for use in this thesis are listed in section 3.4.

3.3 Suitability of the health and disability surveys

In this section we examine the suitability of two types of potentially useful nationwide ABS surveys for this thesis: household surveys and surveys which cover both households and institutions. We compared these two types of surveys because we suspected that earlier findings using a household survey may have been due to a statistical artefact.

These earlier findings suggested that data from household surveys may not be satisfactory when studying health status throughout the life course, because such surveys excluded persons in institutions – such as hospitals, prisons and nursing homes. Walker and Abello (2000) noted that 70+ year old respondents to the ABS's 1995 National Health Survey (NHS) appeared to have better health on average than did younger age groups. Because the reasons for this were unclear at that time, these authors limited their analyses to people aged 70 years or below.

In this section we examine the possibility that this unexpected pattern may have occurred because 70+ year olds who were seriously ill or disabled were in institutions and were thus excluded from the household-based NHS. The findings of this research – carried out for purposes of this thesis – are published in Walker (2002). They are as follows.

We examined two other household surveys: the 1993-94 and 1998-99 Household Expenditure Surveys (HES) conducted by the ABS, but this time health status being indicated by expenditure on pharmaceuticals prescribed by a doctor. The same pattern emerged as in the 1995 NHS that is, in both HES-s, a lower proportion of people aged 75 or over appeared to have spent on prescribed pharmaceuticals – as recorded by respondents over a two-week period - than did in the younger 70+ age group (Figure

3).[11]

Figure 3: **Spenders on prescribed drugs, per cent of the population by age group, 1993-94 and 1998-99**

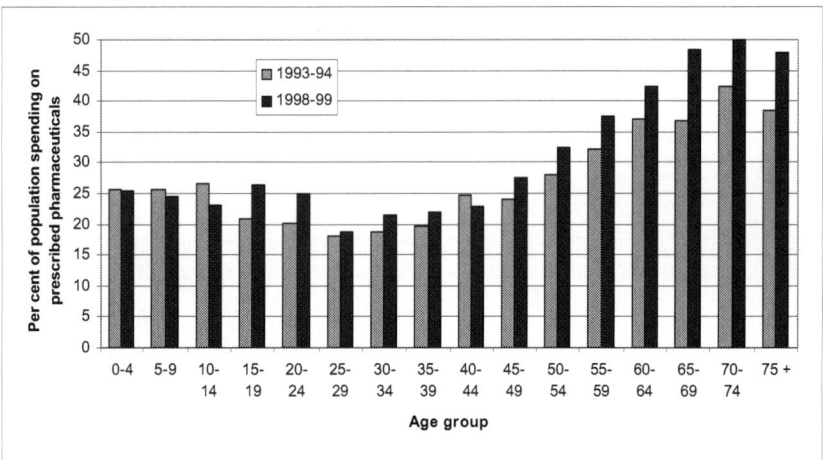

Sources: ABS Household Expenditure Surveys, 1993-94 and 1998-99 - ABS (1995 and 2000b).

While it could be argued that those who survived to age 75 may have had a stronger constitution than the 'younger old', this was not borne out by the statistics reported in the 1998 Disability Survey – a survey which *did include* 5,761 persons in *institutions* as well as 37,580 persons from households (ABS 1999b).

The Disability survey showed that the proportion of Australians with a disability and/or long term illness was increasing steadily well beyond age 70 (Figure 4). Many in the 70+ age group were severely disabled (Appendix 7, Figures A7.2.1 and A7.2.2), with

---

[11] Another interesting pattern in Figure 3 is that in most age groups a higher proportion of persons spent on prescribed drugs in 1998-99 than in 1993-94. This pattern is consistent with the generally upward trend in the number of prescriptions subsidised under Australia's Pharmaceutical Benefits Scheme (a growth rate of close to 3 per cent a year over the period).

around 1% of the disabled with severe restrictions residing in institutions (Table A7.4.2).

Figure 4: **Proportion of population disabled and/or with long-term-illness, 1998**

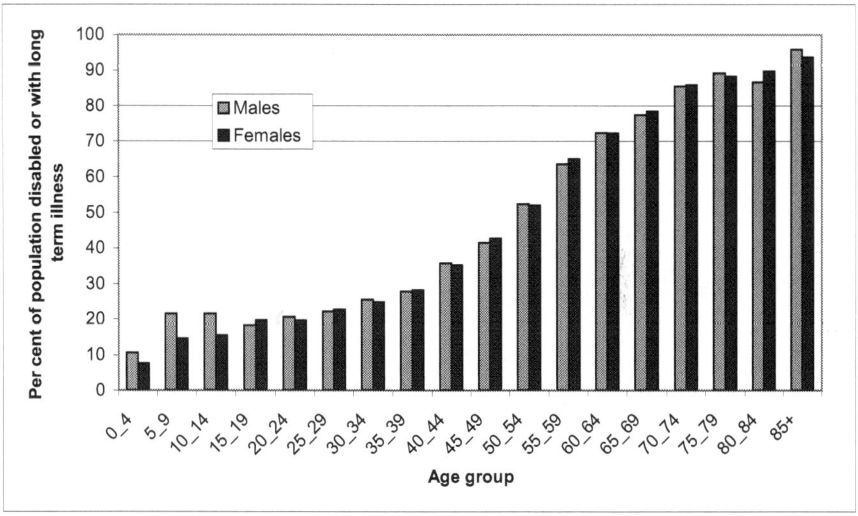

Source: 1998 Disability Survey (ABS 1999a).

Comparing Figures 3 and 4, we conclude that the HES-s significantly underestimate spending on prescribed pharmaceutical in older age groups – probably from age 70 onwards. The problem with excluding people aged over 70 years is that the excluded group accounts for the majority of those who are a year or two away from death[12] – a group of particular importance to studies of lifetime health expenditures and of disability-illness-mortality linkages.

---

[12] In 1996 the life expectancy at birth for Australian men was 75 years, and for women 81 years (Walker 1998). In 2000 life expectancies at birth were 77 years for men and 82 years for women (Dunn et al, 2002). By 2051 these have been projected by the ABS to increase to 81 and 86 years respectively (Walker 1998).

3.4 The data sources chosen

Based on the analyses of section 3.3, the Disability survey was one of the data sources

chosen for building the Health_SES and Health State Transition modules (for data

categories (a) and (c) mentioned in section 3.1), as it is clearly preferable to the

household-based NHS.

As noted in section 3.2, the Disability survey also has linkages to illnesses, in the form

of the 'main disabling condition' variable, as well as information on the severity of

disability. Thus, through the Disability Surveys it is possible to:

- cover the health of not only 0-69 year old Australians, but also of people aged
  70 years or over; and

- establish a link within DYNAMOD between health status and the probability of
  being employed, or the ability of older persons to live independently.

The 1998 Disability survey sample included 15,715 private and special dwellings, with

a 93% response rate. 37,580 persons were interviewed in households and 5,761 in

cared accommodations (ABS 1999b, p.13). Close to 9% of the questionnaires were

incomplete, due mainly to non-response to the question about the annual income of the

family. In the unit record dataset used for purposes of this thesis the records with

income-related non-responses were deleted[13] – with the dataset thus obtained

comprising just over 40,000 observations. Out of the many questions asked on disability

and its severity, the ABS constructed a single 'disabled-or-not' variable (1 if disabled, 0

---

[13] The reason why the option to delete records with income non-responses was chosen, and a
discussion re the extent of bias that may arise from this deletion, are in Appendix 6, section
A6.2.

otherwise), which is the one we used in the analyses reported in Chapters 6. Further details on the Disability survey are in Appendix A2.

Based on the material presented in sections 3.1 and 3.2, the other data source chosen was the AIHW extract of mortality statistics - data category (b) mentioned in section 3.1. These data, by SEIFA quintiles, 5-year age groups, sex, and causes of death (section A2.4.2), were especially purchased for use in this thesis. A special extract was required because the generally available mortality statistics do not have the data disaggregated by all of the above variables. Disaggregation by SEIFA quintiles was essential, because of the thesis objective to study health by SES. Disaggregation by cause of death was also essential because in DYNAMOD the linking of mortality and disability requires - through the equations in section 4.4 - the able-bodied and the disabled to be separately identified.

The AIHW extract covers all deaths over the 1995-97 period and is available to examiners on request. It distinguishes between people who died from external versus non-external causes. When preparing the related input data for DYNAMOD we classified people who died from external causes into the 'able-bodied' group and those who died from non-external causes into the 'disabled' group (section 6.2).

Analysis of the mortality data was carried out using EXCEL, and that of the unit record dataset of the Disability survey – with over 40,000 individual records and 100s of variables – with the SAS programming language.

Chapter 4   Methodology used in developing the Health_SES module

The original dynamic microsimulation model to which the Health_SES and Health State Transition modules were added is a comprehensive model, able to follow individuals in the Australian population from birth to death, through life stages such as education, work, family formation, disability, income patterns and wealth accumulation (section 1.4; Appendix A1).

This Chapter describes the methodology adopted when modelling the Health_SES module (with the methodology for the Health State Transition module being described in section 8.3).

The Chapter first provides an overview of the development of the Health_SES module. Next, it reports on a study – carried out for this thesis - of the relative importance of the factors affecting family income. The aim of this study is to indicate which type of SES measure is most suitable for use in the HEALTH_SES module. Finally, a set of complex equations are presented which link mortality and disability in the dynamic microsimulation model.

Chapters 6 and 7 detail how the Chapter 4 methodology was applied to the preparation of the input data on mortality and disability by age, sex and SES; and to the implementation of the adding a socioeconomic status dimension to DYNAMOD's Base dataset, as well as to the individuals that make up its population in each of the simulation years.

4.1 Overview of the development of the Health_SES module

The section provides an overview of the development of the Health_SES module. It concerns Blocks 1 and 2 and the 'Initialisation' phase of Figure 1 (section 1.5.1), that is:

- imputation of mortality and disability by age, sex and SES in the Base data (Block 1); and

- preparation of the mortality and disability input data (Block 2) for use in the equations section 4.4 ('Initialisation' phase).

Our modelling approach is similar to that in the original model (Antcliff et al, 1996), except that the already complex equations linking disability and mortality now also account for socioeconomic status (section 4.4). Chapters 5, 6 and 7 explain in detail the processes used in this development phase. However, as detailed later in this Chapter, the data sources used to calibrate the equations were updated to 1995-1997 for mortality (AIHW extract described in Appendix, section A2.4.2) and to 1998 for disability (ABS 1999a).

Briefly, to model the health-SES linkages in DYNAMOD we used two indicators of health status (section 4.4):

- mortality rates – which are separately computed for the able-bodied and the disabled, and are linked within DYNAMOD to life expectancy; and

- disability rates – which, apart from being a measure of health status, can also be indicators of quality of life and of health related expenditures.

These two indicators of health status already existed in the original version of DYNAMOD, differentiated by age and sex. However, for purposes of this thesis we needed to also differentiate both these indicators by SES. We did this at the level of quintiles of socioeconomic status.

In the version of DYNAMOD with the Health_SES module added, the linking of mortality and disability by age, sex and SES occurs through the equations described in section 4.4. For example, Figure 5 shows that when a child is born in the model, he/she is allocated a date of death based on historical probabilities of infant mortality for boys and girls, and on his/her parents' socioeconomic status. A mildly or severely disabled new born is allocated an earlier date of death than an able-bodied new born.

Figure 5: **The links modelled between mortality and disability, by SES**

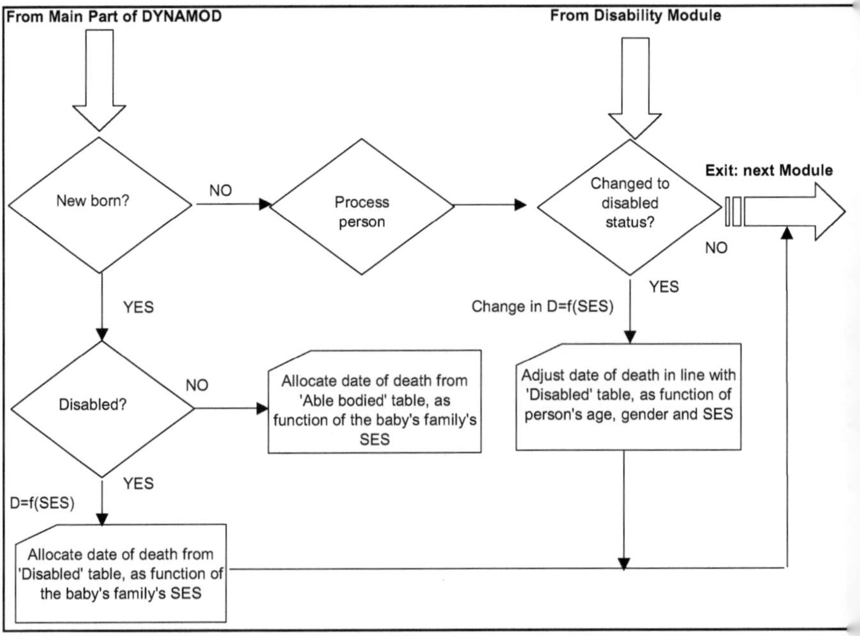

NOTE: D: date of death   SES: family's socioeconomic status.

For all persons in the DYNAMOD population, the date of death and the dates associated with changes in disability status are determined at the beginning of the simulation period ('Initialisation' phase in Figure 1) by survival functions. Such functions determine the probability that a person aged x, whose 'survival' is being studied, will still be alive (or still be able-bodied) at age $x+n$. The equations for these functions are described in section 4.4. The death and disability functions processed at the beginning of the simulation period are only re-evaluated if a change of status from able-bodied to disabled, or vice versa, occurs (Antcliff et al, 1996, pp 21-23). The model has been aligned so that the original mortality rates for the 'able-bodied' and the 'disabled' are maintained throughout the Base (or 'do nothing') simulation, with changes only occurring when better (or worse) health for Australians is simulated.

When considering probabilities of death in later years, the HEALTH_SES module makes use of the increases in life expectancies built into the original model, which were based on predictions published by the Australian Bureau of Statistics. The SES and health states initially allocated by the two new modules to the Base population (sections 7.1 and 8.4) are only modified if a change occurs in a person's health or socioeconomic status in any year of the simulation period. In the model disability affects educational attainment and indirectly, through this link, the employment prospects of the disabled.

We modelled the health-SES link in line with the finding in section 2.4 that, in general, it is low income that causes poor health. That is, health status by SES in the simulation part model is determined *after* the socioeconomic status of a person had been assessed. This assumption regarding the order in which the various life events are processed in DYNAMOD is likely to have a significant impact on the model's results (as is the case with all the other 'ordering' built into any dynamic microsimulation model).

In the Base population of DYNAMOD, disability status was allocated to individuals by socioeconomic status (as well as by age and sex) in line with historically observed patterns (Chapter 7).

4.2 Indicators of health status

This section describes the mortality and disability data used to prepare the input data required by DYNAMOD for the Health_SES module – Block 2 in Figure 1 (section 1.5.1) and for the 'Simulation' phase of that module.

4.2.1 Mortality

As seen in section 2.1, it is common in the literature to use mortality rates and related life expectancies – such as infant mortality or life expectancy at birth - as proxies for health status (World Health Organization, 2000; Mitchell et al, 2000).

However health, as indicated by mortality rates, says nothing about how health problems developed over an individual's life; how these impacted on a person's family or employment prospects; and how that outcome could have been altered through adoption of various interventions by individuals or government. In effect, we know very little from standard statistical collections about the characteristics of people who just died. While such collections tell us when people are likely to die, they say nothing about the quality of their lives prior to death. By simultaneously studying in this thesis *mortality and disability* (section 4.4), we expect to fill some aspects of this knowledge gap.

This section describes the mortality statistics used for estimating the parameters of the section 4.4 equations - with section 4.4.2 detailing the disability data used for parameter estimation purposes in the same set of equations.

The mortality statistics used were especially extracted for this project by the Australian Institute of Health and Welfare (AIHW) from its 1995-97 Mortality Database (Dunn, et al, 2002). Apart from the variables often used in earlier mortality studies – such as age, sex and an index of socioeconomic status based on area of residence – we also obtained data split into two groups based on cause of death. These were 'External' and 'Non-external' causes, which were separately identified so as to be able to distinguish between deaths due to accidents (eg drowning or car crashes) and deaths due to illnesses (eg heart attack). This distinction is important because people dying from external causes are generally much younger than people dying from diseases or old age – hence the former group, although much smaller, is important when estimating the effects of policy changes in terms of 'years of life lost'.

4.2.2 Disability

In search of information on the health related characteristics of Australians, we studied the health and disability statistics available from the Australian Bureau of Statistics. Although these are collected through large cross sectional surveys, it is possible to construct life course patterns by assuming that health patterns for groups with a particular set of demographic and socioeconomic characteristics will remain unchanged over time. While this assumption is adopted as 'default' in the model, allowing for differences in the age-disability profiles – eg across cohorts – could be seen as a possible future improvement.

As discussed in Chapter 3, the ABS's Disability survey was chosen as a key data source for indicating health status. The choices we had were to stay with the 1993-94 survey (used in the original model), or to update the model's Base data using the1998 survey. Because the income variable was a potential candidate for indicating SES, we examined the income related data in both these Disability surveys. We found that the non-response rate to the 'income' question in the 1993-94 survey was much higher than in the 1998 survey. Because of this, we chose the 1998 Disability survey for use in this thesis.

4.3 Key factors affecting family income

Prior to choosing income-based SES indicators for modelling purposes (section 4.4), we investigated which demographic and socioeconomic factors were best able to explain differences in incomes across population groups. To do this we applied regression techniques to the person level data of the 1998 Disability survey (ABS 1999a) – a dataset comprising just over 40,000 records (section 3.4).

The aim was to assess the relative importance of the various factors explaining income. The extent to which disability affected incomes was of particular interest. We used the single 'disabled-or-not' variable (1 if disabled, 0 otherwise) available in the 1998 survey.

For people aged 20 years or above, age, education, employment, occupation and disability were tried as independent variables against the dollar value of equivalent family[14] income, and against the quintile of equivalent[15] family income. Appendix A6 describes the way family income quintiles were computed.

Age (AGE) was a continuous variable taken at the mid-point of the 5-year age groups (2.5 for the 0-5 group, etc... to 85+); disability (DISAB) was (0,1) for all persons classified by the ABS as disabled; education (EDUC) was 'degree or higher', 'professional qualifications' and 'neither of these two'; occupation (OCCUP) was 'managerial/professional', 'semi-professional/clerical' and 'blue collar'; and employment (EMPL), was EMPL=1 if 'employed F/T or P/T' and 0 if unemployed

---

[14] The term 'family', is generally used in this thesis as a proxy for 'income unit'. The ABS (2003, Appendix 1) defines 'income unit' as adults and dependent children within a household whose income is shared.

[15] Appendix 8 describes the equivalence scales used.

(looking for work) or not in the labour force. Note that education, employment and occupation were likely to be correlated with disability and with each other.

Because higher R-squares were obtained with 'quintiles' as the dependent variable than with the dollar value of equivalent family income, we only present the results of multiple linear regression analyses for 'family income quintiles' as the dependent variable. We used the PROC REG function of the SAS programming language. Results are presented in Table 1 both with, and without, the 'disability' variable.

A notable finding is that the R-square values are relatively low, suggesting that there are other important variables affecting 'income'. Another finding is that the regression equations do not change much when the 'disability' variable is removed. Further, all results are highly significant statistically (at the 0.001 level). This is as expected given the large size of the dataset (just over 40,000 records).

Table 1: **Multiple regressions of 'equivalent family income quintile' for persons aged 20 years or over, 1998**

	Coefficient for equation with DISAB	Coefficient for equation without DISAB
	WOMEN	
Intercept	2.29 (0.034) [0.398]	2.26 (0.034) [0.390]
AGE	-0.02 (0.003)	-0.04 (0.003)
EDUC	0.19 (0.011)	0.19 (0.011)
EMPL	0.66 (0.039)	0.71 (0.039)
OCCUP	0.31 (0.017)	0.31 (0.017)
DISAB	-0.07 (0.039)	
	MEN	
Intercept	1.45 (0.041) [0.440]	1.36 (0.040) [0.437]
AGE	0.025 (0.003)	0.018 (0.003)
EDUC	0.24 (0.012)	0.23 (0.012)
EMPL	1.24 (0.037)	1.18 (0.036)
OCCUP	0.26 (0.014)	0.26 (0.014)
DISAB	-0.045 (0.014)	

NOTE: All coefficients were significant at the 0.001 level. Figures in brackets are standard errors and figures in square brackets R-square values.

Based on the magnitude of the related coefficient, 'employment' was the most important variable determining the income quintile to which a person belonged. The sign of the coefficient of 'employment' is positive, as expected, since income is generally higher amongst those employed than amongst people without a job. The coefficient of 'employment' was considerably higher for men than for women.

Of lesser importance were the 'education' and 'occupation' variables, with 'disability' and 'age' being the least important. However, disability is much more important when considering the severely disabled only – see Appendix A7, Figure A7.3.1 and Table A7.4.1. This is one reason why progression of disability from its milder to more severe stages has been chosen for further analysis in this thesis (Chapter 8).

The sign of the disability coefficient was negative for both men and women, which is expected since the incomes of the disabled are generally lower than the incomes of the able-bodied. The sign of the coefficient for age however, while positive for men as expected, was negative for women. This may be because older women in 1998 tended to have very low incomes. The situation is likely to change once the 'baby boomers' replace the current generation of 65+ people, as many women presently in the work force have similar superannuation arrangements to men. Appendix A7 presents further analyses of the health and employment characteristics of Australians.

In summary, important conclusions from the regression analyses are that:

- 'employment' is the single most important variable determining the income quintile to which 20^+ years olds belong (amongst the employment, education, occupation, age and disability variables); and

- having a disability is considerably less important, unless it is 'severe'.

Based on these findings, we chose the 'health-employment' topic for the second application of the enhanced version of DYNAMOD (Chapter 12).[16] That application concerns older Australians, because severe disability is much more prominent in older ages than amongst the young.

4.4 Estimating disability and mortality rates by SES

When estimating disability and mortality rates by SES, the key challenges were: the extension of the complex equations linking mortality and disability in the original version of DYNAMOD by age and sex to a third level of disaggregation - that is by SES as well (sections 4.4.1, 4.4.2, 4.4.3); the finding of data that comprised all the required variables (Chapter 3); and the decision as to which SES indicator to use for disability, given that for mortality only a geographic-area-based SES indicator was available (Chapter 6).

The mortality-disability link is computed using the equations in the original model (Antcliff et al 1996), but with socioeconomic status added as a variable. For computing this link the original (0,1) specification for disability was retained – that is disability=1 if the person is disabled, 0 otherwise.

A summary of the symbols used in the equations described in this section can be found on page xvi. Note that in that summary, as well as throughout this section, the notation refers to disaggregation by age and SES only. In reality, the data was disaggregated by sex and time as well. However in the notation sex, and in most cases time, were omitted for sake of simplicity of presentation. While the variable time t is mentioned in the

---

[16] Had these regressions played a pivotal role in the model building part of the thesis, an effort would have been made to search for the most appropriate specification - eg trying income as both pooled (at quintile level) and non-pooled (at family level) variable; and 'age' as both continuous and dummy variable.

equations used in the simulation phase of DYNAMOD, it was omitted in the equations

arising from survival functions. These latter are used in the initialisation phase of

DYNAMOD (Figure 1, section 1.5.1).[17]

4.4.1   Equations for computing mortality rates: able-bodied and disabled

As noted in section 4.1, in DYNAMOD mortality and disability are linked and, for this

separate mortality data are required for the *able-bodied and the disabled*. Data

limitations required assumptions to be made – the main one being that all deaths from

external causes occurred in the able-bodied population. While this assumption allowed

use of the available data in a complex, mathematical way – see below – it is likely to

lead to over-estimation of mortality rates among the disabled, and underestimation

among the able-bodied. The is because, by ascribing all death from external causes to

the able-bodied, the (unknown) proportion of disabled who die from external causes,

instead of being accounted for among the disabled, are attributed to the able-bodied.

The consequent over and under-estimation is, however, not expected to be large due to a

high proportion of deaths among the elderly arising from chronic diseases - Davis et al

(2002) referred to in section 9.2.

The equations computing mortality rates for these two groups in the 'Initialisation'

phase (Figure 1, section 1.5.1) are described below.

For *the disabled*, the mortality rates - at age x and with SES y - have been

approximated by:

---

[17] In fact, because of our 'default' assumption that health patterns for population groups with a particular set of demographic and socioeconomic characteristics will remain unchanged over time (section 4.2.2), in this thesis the variable t does not affect the mortality and disability related survival functions. It however does affect the individual level *changes* of health states determined in the simulation phase of the model (section 7.2).

$$q^d_{x,y} = \frac{\text{no. of deaths of those aged x in quintile y due to non - external causes}}{\text{disabled population aged x in quintile y}}$$

Similarly, the mortality rates covering deaths form all causes, $q_{x,y}$, were calculated as:

$$q_{x,v} = \frac{\text{total no. of deaths of those aged x in quintile y}}{\text{total population aged x in quintile y}} \qquad \text{Thus,}$$

$$q^d_{x,y} = q_{x,y} \times \frac{\text{no. of deaths (x, y) due to non - external causes}}{\text{total no. of deaths of those aged (x, y)}} \times \frac{\text{total population (x, y)}}{\text{disabled population aged (x, y)}}$$

If $p_{x,y}$ is the prevalence of disability at age x then

$$\frac{\text{total population aged (x, y)}}{\text{disabled population aged (x, y)}} = \frac{1}{p_{x,y}}$$

Since the prevalence $p_{x,y}$ is known, we only need to compute the proportion of deaths due to non-external causes to obtain an estimate for $q^d_{x,y}$.

The equation for *the able bodied* population is similar, except that the mortality statistics are for external causes and the prevalence is for the able bodied:

$$\frac{\text{total population aged (x, y)}}{\text{able bodied population aged (x, y)}} = \frac{1}{1 - p_{x,y}}$$

4.4.2 Equations linking disability and mortality by SES

This section describes the way disability and mortality are linked - within each age, sex and SES cell - in the 'Initialisation' phase in Figure 1 (section 1.5.1). Briefly, disability decrements rates are derived using standard multiple decrement techniques (Antcliff et 1996). Within each cell, the able bodied population is subject to exits due to death and entrants due to recovery, while the disabled population is subject to exits due to death and recovery and entrants due to disability onsets.

The following steps have been taken to build up a double decrement rate for both mortality and disability.

(a) definitions

Let:

$l_{x,y}^a$ be the number in able-bodied population aged x, with family SES quintile y

$l_{x,y}^d$ be the number in the disabled population aged x, with family SES quintile y

$R_{x,y}$ be the number of recoveries aged x, with family SES quintile y

$D_{x,y}$ be the number of people becoming disabled, aged x, SES quintile y

$q_{x,y}^a$ is the mortality rate for the able-bodied population

$q_{x,y}^d$ the mortality rate for the disabled population

(b) equations linking the able-bodied and disabled mortality rates

In calculating independent death rates for the able-bodied population, those initially exposed to risk are given by:

$$E_{x,y}^a = l_{x,y}^a + \tfrac{1}{2}.R_{x,y} - \tfrac{1}{2}.D_{x,y} \qquad \text{and similarly for the disabled population}$$

$$E_{x,y}^d = l_{x,y}^d - \tfrac{1}{2}.R_{x,y} + \tfrac{1}{2}.D_{x,y}$$

Then making use of $q_{x,y}^a$ and $q_{x,y}^d$ we have

$$E_{x,y}^a.q_{x,y}^a + E_{x,y}^d.q_{x,y}^d = E_{x,y}.q_{x,y} \qquad \text{where } E_{x,y} \text{ is the initial exposed risk for all persons}$$

within that particular SES quintile, y. Thus, the equation linking the able-bodied and disabled mortality rates is:

$$q_{x,y}^d = \frac{\left(l_{x,y}^a + l_{x,y}^d\right)q_{x,y} - \left(l_{x,y}^a + \tfrac{1}{2}.R_{x,y} - \tfrac{1}{2}.D_{x,y}\right)q_{x,y}^a}{l_{x,y}^d - \tfrac{1}{2}.R_{x,y} + \tfrac{1}{2}.D_{x,y}} \qquad (1)$$

(c) Size and linking of the able bodied and disabled populations

Equations (2) and (3) below estimate the number of persons in the able bodied and disabled populations.

$$l^a_{(x+1),y} = l^a_{x,y} - D_{x,y} + R_{x,y} - \left(l^a_{x,y} + \tfrac{1}{2}.R_{x,y} - \tfrac{1}{2}.D_{x,y}\right)q^a_{x,y} \tag{2}$$

$$l^d_{(x+1),y} = l^d_{x,y} - R_{x,y} + D_{x,y} - \left(l^d_{x,y} - \tfrac{1}{2}.R_{x,y} + \tfrac{1}{2}.D_{x,y}\right)q^d_{x,y} \tag{3}$$

The able bodied and disabled populations can be related at any point in time using the prevalence rate for the appropriate age within the SES quintile being studied. Equation (4) links the able-bodied and disabled population as:

$$l^d_{(x+1),y} = l^a_{(x+1),y} . \frac{P_{(x+1),y}}{1 - P_{(x+1),y}} \tag{4}$$

which, upon substituting from expressions (A.1), (A.2), (A.3), gives for each SES quintile:

$$l^d_x - R_x + D_x - \left(l^d_x - \tfrac{1}{2}.R_x + \tfrac{1}{2}.D_x\right)\frac{\left(l^a_x + l^d_x\right)q_x - \left(l^a_x + \tfrac{1}{2}.R_x - \tfrac{1}{2}.D_x\right)q^a_x}{l^d_x - \tfrac{1}{2}.R_x + \tfrac{1}{2}.D_x} = \frac{P_{x+1}}{1-P_{x+1}}\left(l^a_x - D_x + R_x - \left(l^a_x + \tfrac{1}{2}.R_x - \tfrac{1}{2}.D_x\right)q^a_x\right)$$

This equation is linear in $D_{x,y}$ and therefore can be solved as described below.

(d) Building the double decrement table for death and disability

From the above equation the number of people becoming disabled, $D_{x,y}$ can be expressed as:

$$D_{x,y} = \frac{P_{(x+1),y}.l^a_{x,y} + R_{x,y} - q^a_{x,y}.\left(l^a_{x,y} + \tfrac{1}{2}.R_{x,y}\right) - \left(1 - P_{(x+1),y}\right)\left\{l^d_{x,y}.\left(1 - q_{x,y}\right) - l^a_{x,y}.q_{x,y}\right\}}{1 - \tfrac{1}{2}.q^a_{x,y}} \tag{5}$$

For any given values of $R_{x,y}$ this formula can be used to build up a *double decrement table for death and disability*. Because data are not available for $R_{x,y}$, values for this variable have been chosen based on the same assumptions as in (Antcliff et al 1996, p. 115). These assumptions are: (i) $D_{x,y}$ remains positive for all ages within the SES quintile being studied; and (ii) $D_{x,y}$ starts at 4% of the disabled population at age 0, increases to 15% of the disabled population over the age range 11 to 40 and then gradually declines to zero by age 94. Independent rates of increments due to disability and recovery, $r_{x,y}$ and $d_{x,y}$ were then calculated – as in Antcliff et al (1996) - from $R_{x,y}$ and $D_{x,y}$ using the relationship:

$$r_{x,y} = \frac{R_{x,y}}{l_{x,y}^d + \frac{1}{2}.D_{x,y} - \frac{1}{2}.\theta_{x,y}^d} \tag{6}$$

$$d_{x,y} = \frac{D_{x,y}}{l_{x,y}^a + \frac{1}{2}.R_{x,y} - \frac{1}{2}.\theta_{x,y}^a} \tag{7}$$

$\theta_{x,y}^a$ being number of deaths in the able–bodied population aged x with SES quintile y; and

$\theta_{x,y}^d$ the number of deaths in the disabled population aged x with SES quintile y.

4.4.3   *Equations for deriving future mortality rates*

This section describes how changes in future mortality rates are modelled in the 'Initialisation' and 'Simulation' phases of Figure 1 (section 1.5.1). Allowing for improvements in life expectancies in DYNAMOD is important, given the potential length of the simulation period. To do this, within each age, sex and SES quintile cell, the likelihood that people live longer (on average) in later years of the simulation period than in earlier ones, is programmed in. Also programmed is a parameter, by age, sex and SES quintile cell, which determines the proportion of the improvement allocated to able-bodied population - the rest being experienced by the disabled.

In the original model, the improvements in total mortality rates by age and sex follow the assumptions implicit in published ABS population projections. Since there are no data on such improvements by SES quintile as well, we assumed that the improvements are distributed in a proportional fashion across SES quintiles. As a default, we assumed that, within each SES quintile, the able-bodied population has improvements in mortality rates equivalent to half of the improvements in total mortality rates in that quintile. These default assumptions can be changed by the user, as required.

The independent rates of recovery and disability derived using the methodology outlined in Antcliff et al (1996) have been assumed to remain unchanged in the enhanced version of the model. However, alternative assumptions about future trends in onset of disability and recovery could be incorporated in future.

Because mortality rates change over time - due to use of the life expectancy 'improvement' factors - the computations can no longer be confined to age, sex and SES cells. The variable t also becomes relevant, indicating the simulation year.

We assumed that:

$$r_{x,y,t} = r_{x,y} \qquad \text{for all t; and}$$

$$d_{x,y,t} = d_{x,y} \qquad \text{for all t .}$$

The mortality rate for the total population evolves over time as:

$$q_{x,y,t} = q_{x,y,0} \times \prod_{i=1}^{t} \left[1 + \frac{\delta(x,y,i)}{100} \right]$$

where $\delta(x,y,i)$ is the percentage change in the total mortality rate, within quintile y, in year i and at age x. Note that $\delta(x,y,i) \le 0$ for all x and i.

The mortality rate for the able-bodied becomes:

$$q^a_{x,y,t} = q^a_{x,y,0} \times \prod_{i=1}^{t}\left[1+0.5\frac{\delta(x,y,i)}{100}\right]$$

To calculate $q^d_{x,y,t}$ we made use of the following equations:

$$\theta^a_{x,y,t} = \left(l^a_{x,y,t} - \tfrac{1}{2}.D_{x,y,t} + \tfrac{1}{2}.R_{x,y,t}\right)q^a_{x,y,t} \tag{8}$$

$$D_{x,y,t} = \left(l^a_{x,y,t} - \tfrac{1}{2}.\theta^a_{x,y,t} + \tfrac{1}{2}.R_{x,y,t}\right)d_{x,y} \tag{9}$$

$$\theta^d_{x,y,t} = \left(l^d_{x,y,t} - \tfrac{1}{2}.R_{x,y,t} + \tfrac{1}{2}.D_{x,y,t}\right)q^d_{x,y,t} \tag{10}$$

$$R_{x,y,t} = \left(l^d_{x,y,t} - \tfrac{1}{2}.\theta^d_{x,y,t} + \tfrac{1}{2}.D_{x,y,t}\right)r_{x,y} \tag{11}$$

and equation (1), giving:

$$q^d_{x,y,t} = \frac{\left(l^a_{x,y,t} + l^d_{x,y,t}\right)q_{x,y} - \left(l^a_{x,y,t} + \tfrac{1}{2}.R_{x,y,t} - \tfrac{1}{2}.D_{x,y,t}\right)q^a_{x,y,t}}{l^d_{x,t} - \tfrac{1}{2}.R_{x,t} + \tfrac{1}{2}.D_{x,t}} \tag{12}$$

Equations (8) to (11) may be solved for $R_{x,y,t}$ and $D_{x,y,t}$, giving the following expressions:

$$R_{x,y,t} = \frac{r_{x,y}.\left(1 - \tfrac{1}{2}.q^d_{x,y,t}\right)\left\{l^d_{x,y,t}.\left(1 - \tfrac{1}{4}.d_{x,y}.q^a_{x,y,t}\right) + \tfrac{1}{2}.d_{x,y}.l^a_{x,y,t}.\left(1 - \tfrac{1}{2}q^a_{x,y,t}\right)\right\}}{\left(1 - \tfrac{1}{4}.r_{x,y}.q^d_{x,y,t}\right)\left(1 - \tfrac{1}{4}.d_{x,y}.q^a_{x,y,t}\right) - \tfrac{1}{2}.r_{x,y}.d_{x,y}.\left(1 - \tfrac{1}{2}.q^a_{x,y,t}\right)\left(1 - \tfrac{1}{2}.q^d_{x,y,t}\right)} \tag{13}$$

$$D_{x,y,t} = \frac{d_{x,y}.\left(1 - \tfrac{1}{2}.q^a_{x,y,t}\right)\left\{l^a_{x,y,t}.\left(1 - \tfrac{1}{4}.r_{x,y}.q^d_{x,y,t}\right) + \tfrac{1}{2}.r_{x,y}.l^d_{x,y,t}.\left(1 - \tfrac{1}{2}q^d_{x,y,t}\right)\right\}}{\left(1 - \tfrac{1}{4}.r_{x,y}.q^d_{x,y,t}\right)\left(1 - \tfrac{1}{4}.d_{x,y}.q^a_{x,y,t}\right) - \tfrac{1}{2}.r_{x,y}.d_{x,y}.\left(1 - \tfrac{1}{2}.q^a_{x,y,t}\right)\left(1 - \tfrac{1}{2}.q^d_{x,y,t}\right)} \tag{14}$$

Since $q^d_{x,y,t}$ will change only slowly over time, we can use – as in Antcliff et al (1996) –

$q^d_{x,y,t-1}$ as a first approximation to $q^d_{x,y,t}$ in equations (13) and (14) and then substitute

the values for $R_{x,y,t}$ and $D_{x,y,t}$ in equation (12) to get a value for $q^d_{x,y,t}$. Through a process of iteration we can converge to the exact solution for $q^d_{x,y,t}$ We then use the following expressions to generate the $l_{x,y}$ values for the next year in the decrement table:

$$l^a_{x+1,y,t+1} = l^a_{x,y,t}.\left(1 - q^a_{x,y,t} - d_{x,y}\right) + l^d_{x,y,t}.r_{x,y}$$

$$l^d_{x+1,y,t+1} = l^d_{x,y,t}.\left(1 - q^d_{x,y,t} - r_{x,y}\right) + l^a_{x,y,t}.d_{x,y}$$

and thus recursively derive disabled mortality rates, by SES quintile, for all ages and all years of the simulation.

Within each SES quintile, the probability of a disabled person aged x at time t still being alive at age $x+n$ is then:

$$\left(1 - q^d_{x,y,t}\right)\left(1 - q^d_{x+1,y,t+1}\right)\left(1 - q^d_{x+2,y,t+2}\right)...\left(1 - q^d_{x+n-1,y,t+n-1}\right) = \prod_{i=0}^{n-1}\left(1 - q^d_{x+i,y,t+i}\right)$$

and similarly for an able-bodied person the survival function is:

$$\left(1 - q^a_{x,y,t}\right)\left(1 - q^a_{x+1,y,t+1}\right)\left(1 - q^a_{x+2,y,t+2}\right)...\left(1 - q^a_{x+n-1,y,t+n-1}\right) = \prod_{i=0}^{n-1}\left(1 - q^a_{x+i,y,t+i}\right)$$

We calculate the expected date of death each time a person becomes disabled or recovers by generating a random number p and finding n such that, for a person becoming disabled at time t:

$$\prod_{i=1}^{n}\left(1 - q^d_{x+i,y,t+i}\right) < p < \prod_{i=1}^{n-1}\left(1 - q^d_{x+i,y,t+i}\right)$$

The date of death is then:

$$12.n + INT\left[12.\left\{p - \prod_{i=1}^{n}\left(1 - q^d_{x+i,y,t+i}\right)\right\}\right]$$

months away from time t.

Antcliff et al (1996, pp 1) describe the mechanisms programmed into DYNAMOD for storing and using these expected times of death during the simulation phase (Block 4 in Figure 1, section 1.5.1).

4.5 Conclusion

In this Chapter we showed that, for Australians aged 20 years or more, the key determinant of the income-based socioeconomic status is whether they have a job – with education, occupation and age being less important. Health, as indicated by disability, was considerably less important in explaining people's incomes - and thus their income-based SES - unless disability was associated with severe restrictions in core activities (section 4.3). These findings are consistent with those reported in the literature (sections 2.3, 2.4).

A novel feature of the approach adopted in this Chapter is a move away from the traditional mortality-based indicator of health, towards a methodology able to account for disability over the life course, together with its eventual impact on mortality. In essence, we re-focussed the analyses toward 'what quality of life people will have while they are alive' from the more traditional 'how long will people live for' approach.

In addition, we accounted for the health-mortality relationship by SES, as well as by the traditional age-sex variables generally considered in the literature. This was achieved through a complex set of equations, described in sections 4.4.1, 4.4.2, and 4.4.3.

Chapter 5 Comparing geographic-area-based and individual-based SES indicators

This Chapter addresses the question of which type of SES indicator is most appropriate for the studies of health inequalities planned for this thesis. This question is relevant in cases where there is a choice between geographic area-based and individuals' income-based indicators of SES. To the author's knowledge, this issue has not to date been published in the literature.

The study presented in this Chapter reports on new research, carried out for this thesis, analysing nationwide survey data in innovative ways. It is shortly to be published in Walker and Becker (2005).

In studies of health inequalities different strands of the literature tend to use different indicators of SES. The traditional approach is based on cross-sectional analyses, using mortality as the indicator of health and a geographic-area based index as a measure of socioeconomic status – Acheson (1998); Marmot (1986); Pamuk et al (1998); Turrell and Mathers (2000, 2001, 2002).

In some cases data constraints mean that only one type of indicator is available and in such cases researchers have no alternative but to use that type. In situations where several types of indicators could be constructed, some limited guidance can obtained from the 'ecological fallacy' literature in relation to choice of aggregate versus individual-based data in regression analyses for individual-level models – Robinson (1950). Jargowsky (2003) found that different estimates were obtained at different levels of aggregation. The level of aggregation is an important issue for this Chapter, because the geographic area-based indicators - which allocate the *same* SES to each person living in a particular area – operate at an aggregate level.

In this Chapter we compare the use, in health inequality studies, of the geographically based Socioeconomic Index for Areas (SEIFA) with two individual-based SES indicators able to account for family income and size. These indicators were chosen because of their relevance to the model-building part of the thesis. Inequalities in disability prevalences by SES are measured using age-standardised rate ratios. Logistic regression is used to determine which type of SES measure is a better predictor of the observed disability prevalences. The data source used is the 1998 Disability survey (ABS 1999a), with the single 'disabled-or-not' variable (1 if disabled, 0 otherwise) – section 4.3.

5.1 Aims of analyses

Studies of mortality are important because they reflect duration of life. They are also convenient because data are often available and complete. As seen in Chapter 1, studies of disability are also valuable because they reflect quality of life, can be studied throughout the life course, and are associated with mortality. Furthermore, for the generally available mortality data the only information from which deceased persons' socioeconomic status can be imputed is their last residential address. The related geographic-area based SES indexes result in all persons living in a particular area being allocated the same socioeconomic status. Relying on such indexes in studies of health inequalities is recognised to have significant limitations – HM Treasury (1999); ABS (2001a and 1998c); McCracken (2001).

In this Chapter we use the same population to study the association of disability with each of three SES indexes, one traditional geographic-area-based index and two individual-based SES indicators. Specifically we consider whether:

(a) the three types of SES measures produce similar estimates of health inequalities, as indicated by observed disability data; and

(b) whether some SES indicators are better predictors of a person being disabled than others.

Objective (b) is intended to indicate levels of support for each SES index in the event that their estimates of health inequalities differ.

5.2 Indicators of health and socioeconomic status

The measure chosen for health status in this study was disability because it allows greater consideration of the important life course and quality of life implications of health than does mortality (section 4.2). We expressed disability as *rate per 100 population* (i.e. percent disabled), computed for five broad age groups: 0-19, 20-39, 40-59, 60-69 and 70+.

As measures of socioeconomic status we considered three different types of indicator:

- the geographic-area-based SEIFA index[18] – Appendix A3;

- an indicator based on individuals' family income; and

- an individual-based indicator accounting for both family income and family size.

---

[18] Based on their residential address, this index was applied by the ABS to respondents in the Disability survey at the level of the smallest area available, the Census Collection District. Glover et al (2004) and Hyndman et al (1995) have shown that, compared with CD level analyses, studies at the larger postcode and Statistical Local Area levels understated health differentials by SES.

Of the five SEIFA indexes available in the 1998 Disability Survey (Appendix A3), we

chose the Index of Relative Socioeconomic Disadvantage because it is the one

developed for studying socioeconomic inequalities. This index is attached, in the form

of deciles, to each respondent in the 1998 Disability survey. It is based on the

geographic location of their residential addresses. We aggregated these deciles to

quintiles so that, when weighted (using the survey weights), each SES quintile based on

the SEIFA comprised 20% of the Australian population – Quintile 1 (Q1) the 20% most

disadvantaged and Quintile 5 (Q5) the 20% least disadvantaged.

From the variables available in the Disability Survey we constructed two *individual-

based SES indicators* that account for family income and family size. The importance of

using SES indicators that reflect the economic resources available to families is widely

recognised – ABS (2001a, 2003a and b); Saunders (1996). The two individual-based

SES indicators constructed for this study are:

    Income   Inc = total weekly cash income of family

    Equivalent Income   EqInc = Inc/ (Equivalence scale factor)

The Equivalence scale factor was computed at the family level using the modified

OECD scale – giving a weights of 1 for the first adult in the family; 0.5 for each

subsequent adult; and 0.3 for each dependent child (Appendix A8). Data permitting,

the EqInc indicator is often preferred because – as noted above - it is a more appropriate

indicator of the economic resources available to a family than the Inc indicator (ABS

2003b).

A limitation of these Inc and EqInc measures is that they do not account for the wealth

that families have - because 'wealth' is not a variable in the Disability survey. One

effect of this is that older people may be allocated to a lower socioeconomic quintile

than if wealth had also been accounted for.

5.3 Do the three types of SES measures produce similar estimates of health inequalities?

When studying the issues under objective (a), health inequality was expressed as the disability *rate ratio* of SES quintile 1 (Q1) to SES quintile 5 (Q5) – an internationally accepted measure of inequality, widely used in health and epidemiological research (Draper et al 2004).[19] Inequality estimates for the total population were age standardised to the 1998 Australian population by SEIFA quintile (Appendix A10). We also carried out tests of statistical significance on the estimated inequalities. A standard test for the comparison of proportions was used to test the hypothesis that the disability *rate ratio* was equal to 1 (Appendix A11).

Prior to tabulating health inequalities in terms of rate ratios we present, for each of the three SES indicators, charts that illustrate differences in estimates of health inequalities across the SEIFA, Inc and EqInc measures.

5.4 Are some SES indicators better predictors of a person being disabled than others?

In studying the issue under objective (b) we fitted logistic regression models – Lee (1974); McCullagh and Nelder (1989) - to the 1998 Disability survey dataset to estimate the probability that an individual is disabled, using the SES indicators as predictors. Other predictors were age and sex. Age and SES were categorical variables. Specifically, we assumed that individual i, with explanatory variables denoted by x_i, has response probability $p_i = \text{prob(disability} = 1 \mid x_i)$ given by $e^{\eta}/(1 + e^{\eta})$, where

$$\eta = \mu + \text{Age}_j + \beta^* \text{Sex} + \text{SES}_k$$

---

[19] While the Gini coefficient is also an often used measure of inequality, it was not chosen for this thesis because the results it produces are less comprehensible to the average intelligent reader than those of the Q1/Q5 measure.

Age_j is the parameter for the age category of the individual (5-year groupings from 0-4 to 70+). We used age as a categorical variable to avoid assumptions about the relationship between age and disability.

Sex is 0 for males and 1 for females.

SES_k is the parameter for the SES quintile of the individual.

Note that Age_j and SES_k do not require coefficients in the above equation because they are parameters reflecting categorical variables.

5.5 Results

5.5.1   Inequalities in health by SEIFA – Objective (a)

Figure 6 shows the disability rates in the 1998 survey by SES and age for the SEIFA, Inc and EqInc indicators. Regardless of the type of SES measure chosen, the within-age-group disability rates are consistently higher for people in the poorest quintile than in any other quintile. This is in line with the 'ecological fallacy' literature mentioned earlier in the Chapter which concluded that different levels of aggregation led to different model estimates - Jargowsky (2003).

This is broadly in line with the findings of earlier studies - Turrell and Mathers (2000); ABS (2003b); Saunders (1996). However, care must be taken not to automatically interpret these results as 'low SES causes individuals to be more susceptible to disabilities', because in some instances it is the disability that causes SES to become low (section 2.4).

Figure 6 also shows that the within age-group health inequalities (i.e. the Q1 to Q5 differences) are consistently greater when estimated with the individual-based SES indicators than with the SEIFA.

Figure 6: **Proportion disabled by age and type of SES indicator***

SEIFA quintiles

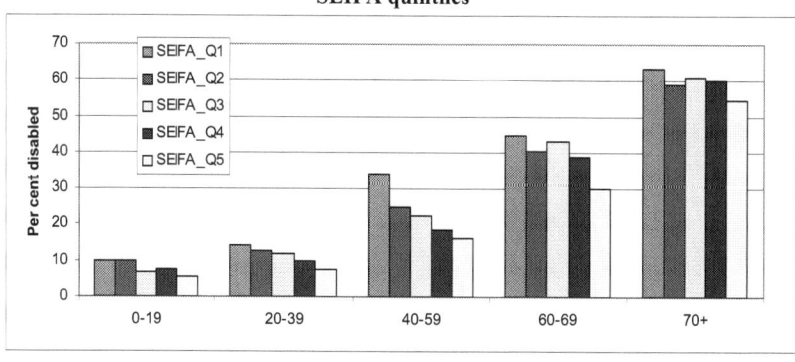

Income quintiles

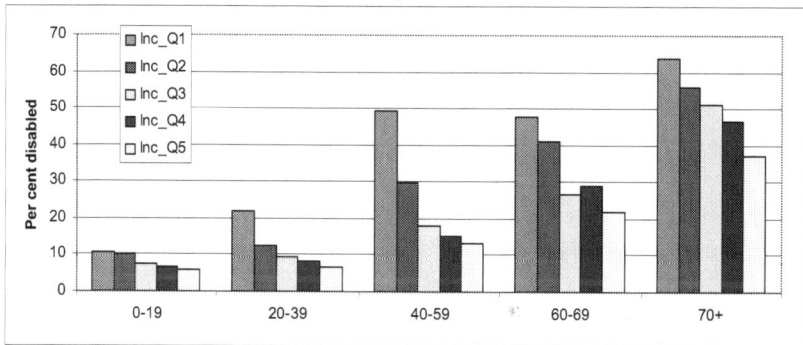

Equivalent Income quintiles

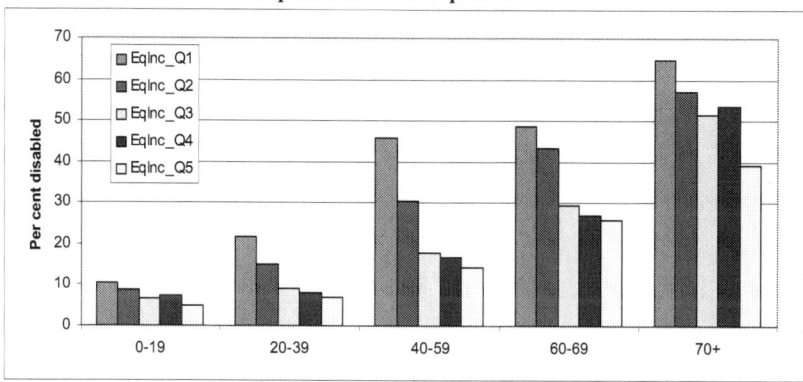

* Q1 is the poorest and Q5 the richest SES quintile.
Data source: 1998 Disability Survey (ABS 1999a), weighted cross tabulations

When we chart the age-standardised disability rates by SES only,[20] the individual-based

indicators once again show a markedly greater difference in disability rates between

rich and poor than does the SEIFA (Figure 7). A noteworthy feature of Figure 7 is that,

for the Inc and EqInc indicators, the familiar near-linear downward SES gradient

reported in much of the SEIFA-based literature is replaced by a curved relationship,

with greater differences in disability rates between the two extreme SES quintiles than

with the SEIFA.

Figure 7: **Proportion disabled by type of SES indicator,* 1998**

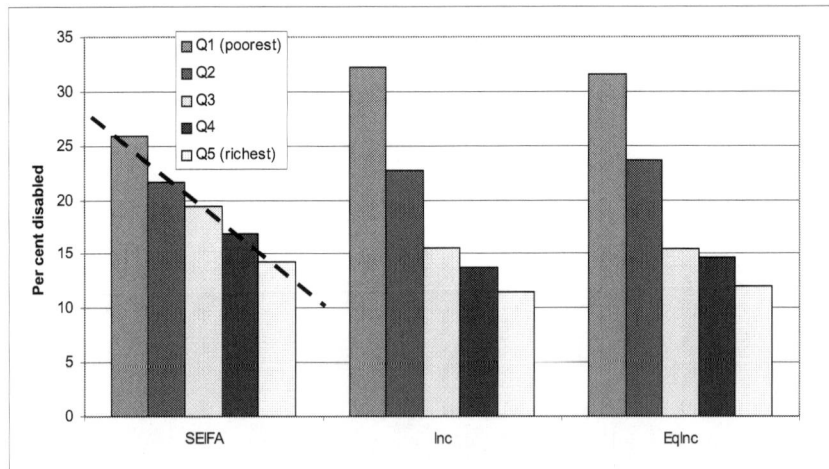

* Age standardised to the 1998 population by SEIFA quintile – see Appendix A10.
Data source: 1998 Disability Survey (ABS 1999a), weighted cross tabulations

To address Objective (a) more specifically we present health inequality estimates for the

SEIFA, Inc and EqInc indicators using Q1/Q5 as inequality measure – – that is, the ratio

of the disability rate of the poorest SES quintile to that of the richest (Table 2).

---

[20] Inequality estimates for the total population were age standardised to the 1998 Australian
population (section 5.3 and Appendix A10).

Table 2 shows that, within each age group, the proportion disabled in Q1 in 1998 was

considerably higher than that in Q5.

Table 2: **Differences in the proportion disabled by age and type of socioeconomic status indicator, 1998**

	Proportion disabled		Q1/Q5
	Q1	Q5	
	%	%	Rate ratio^
SEIFA quintiles			
0 - 19 yo	9.7	5.6	1.74
20 – 39 yo	14.2	7.7	1.85
40 – 59 yo	34.2	16.3	2.09
60 – 69 yo	44.6	30.2	1.48
70+ yo	63.2	54.6	1.16
Total*	25.9	14.3	1.82
Income quintiles			
0 - 19 yo	10.5	5.7	1.84
20 – 39 yo	21.7	6.8	3.20
40 – 59 yo	49.2	13.3	3.71
60 – 69 yo	47.6	21.9	2.18
70+ yo	63.7	37.0	1.72
Total*	32.2	11.4	2.82
Equivalent Income quintiles			
0 - 19 yo	10.5	4.9	2.12
20 – 39 yo	21.8	7.1	3.06
40 – 59 yo	45.7	14.5	3.15
60 – 69 yo	48.8	25.8	1.89
70+ yo	64.7	39.3	1.64
Total*	31.6	12.1	2.61

* Totals are age standardised to the 1998 population by SEIFA quintile – see Appendix A10.
^ All estimates of rate ratios are significant at $p<0.001$ except for the 70+ age group with Income as SES indicator, which is significant at $p<0.01$ –see Appendix A11.

Data Source: 1998 Disability Survey (ABS 1999a), weighted cross tabulations.

For example, with the SEIFA, the proportion disabled amongst 0-19 year olds in Q1

was 74% greater than that amongst 0-19 year olds in Q5. As expected - when using such

a large dataset - the differences shown in the Table are statistically highly significant

($p<0.001$ or $p<0.01$).

Table 2 quantifies the differences in health inequalities that were illustrated visually in Figures 6 and 7. For example the inequality indicated by the age-standardised rate ratio for all age groups is 1.82 with the SEIFA, compared with 2.82 and 2.61 with Inc and EqInc respectively (Table 2). In other words, while with the individual-based indicators the poorest 20% of Australians were found to have a disability rate that was more than 150% greater than that of the richest 20%, the SEIFA only measured that difference as 82%.

5.5.2   Comparing the predictive ability by type of SES indicator – Objective (b)

The results of fitting a logistic regression model to the indicator of disability are summarised in Table 3. As expected, age is the most important factor explaining disability (a likelihood ratio chi-square value of 14887 on 15 degrees of freedom). Adding the variable 'sex' improves the fit significantly ($\chi2 = 23$ on 1 df, $p<0.001$). Adding the SEIFA indicator to the age and sex factors improves the fit further ($\chi2 = 259$ on 4 df).

Table 3: **Logistic regressions – SES indicators as predictors of disability**

Predictors included	Likelihood Ratio Chi-square (df)*		% concordant
age		14887 (15)	80.7
age, sex	wrt age	23 (1)	81.9
age, sex, SEIFA	wrt age,sex	259 (4)	83.1
age, sex, Inc	wrt age,sex	2157 (4)	84.9
age, sex, EqInc	wrt age,sex	2113 (4)	84.8

* degree of freedom in brackets;   **NOTE**: all results are significant at $p<0.0001$.

Data source: Logistic regression analyses using the 1998 Disability Survey (ABS 1999a), unweighted

An important finding is that the likelihood ratio χ^2 for the Inc and EqInc indicators is an order of magnitude greater than that of the SEIFA (2157 and 2113, compared with 259). This suggests that the individual-based Inc or EqInc indicators have considerably better explanatory powers than the geographic-area-based SEIFA. This conclusion is also reflected by the '% concordant' statistic reproduced in Table 3.

5.6 Discussion

Although the differences in health inequalities reflected by the various SES indicators are anticipated, the magnitudes of the differences between the SEIFA and the Inc/EqInc indicators are noteworthy. Our findings mean that 'family income'-based SES measures are substantially better identifiers of individuals with a disability than the geographic area based SEIFA.

The EqInc index does not perform quite as well as the 'family income' indicator, as indicated by its slightly less '% concordant' statistic in Table 2 (84.8% compared with 84.9%). This suggests that the weights given to 'other adults' and 'children' are not optimal in terms of making EqInc the preferred predictor of disability.

Table 3 shows that disability prevalence differs significantly between males and females. However, after adjusting for age, sex is a substantially weaker predictor of disability than each of the SES indicators.

Age is by far the best predictor of disability. This makes it extremely important to adjust for age – as is done through age standardisation in this study - when comparing the SES indicators as predictors. When age is not included in the logistic regression the advantage of Inc (and EqInc) as a predictor, over SEIFA, appears much greater. However, this is due to the fact that Inc (and EqInc) is associated with age much more strongly than is the SEIFA. Indeed, the ABS cautions that it does not consider the age structure of the population when it develops the SEIFA indexes (Appendix A3). Figure 8 shows the effect of this, with the 'implied' age distributions across SEIFA quintiles being remarkably stable, compared with the distributions across the Inc or EqInc quintiles.

The relative stability across SEIFA quintiles may stem from the fact that the SEIFA allocates the same SES to all persons residing in a given geographic area.

Another explanation of the differences in age distribution seen in Figure 8 is that, unlike the 'family income'–based indicators, the SEIFA does not account for the known life-course-related differences in SES – i.e that young adults tend to start with low SES, progress to higher socioeconomic quintiles by middle age and generally experience a decline in their socioeconomic status after retirement.

5.7 Conclusions and possible future improvements

In the original research described in this Chapter, estimates of health inequalities obtained with the SEIFA were found to be considerably lower than those obtained with the income-based individual-level SES indicators. With the SEIFA, the proportion disabled amongst the most disadvantaged 20% of Australians was estimated to be 82% higher than amongst the most advantaged 20%, compared with over 150% with the individual-based SES measures. Also, the individual-based indicators were considerably better predictors of observed disability status than the SEIFA.

Figure 8: **Age distribution within SES quintiles, Disability Survey, 1998**

SEIFA quintiles

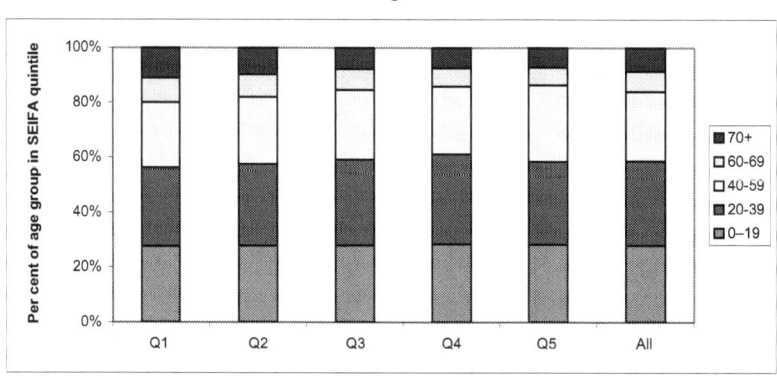

Income quintiles

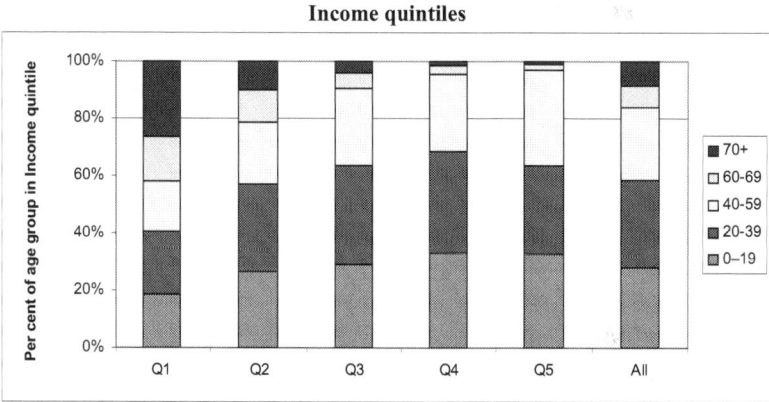

Equivalent Income quintiles

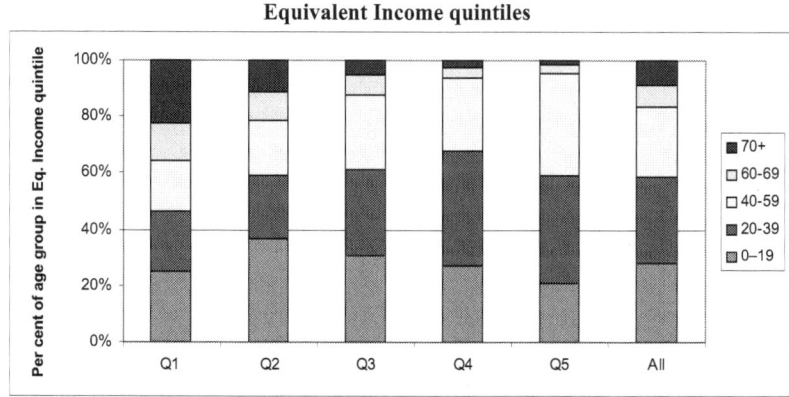

Quintile 1 is most disadvantaged; Quintile 5 is least disadvantaged
Source: 1998 Disability Survey (ABS, 1999a), weighted cross tabulations.

5.7.1   Conclusions

An important conclusion is that estimates of health inequalities can vary considerably with the indicator of SES chosen. Another conclusion is that he health-SES patterns traditionally reported in the mortality-based literature no longer hold with income/wealth based indicators of health, and when population ageing is accounted for.

A further conclusion is that an individual-level SES indicator - such as one based on family income – is more appropriate for studies of income inequalities than a geographic area-based index, such as the SEIFA. This is because age, which was found to be the single most important factor affecting disability, is not a variable that is considered by the ABS when it develops its SEIFA indexes. By comparison, the individual-based indicators are able to fully reflect the variations in socioeconomic status that exist amongst people of different ages living in a particular area.

In view of the above, and of the 'health inequalities' focus of this thesis, we concluded that - whenever possible - the individual income-based indicators of SES should be used for purposes of this project.

5.7.2   Possible future improvements

It would be useful to develop income-based SES indicators similar to the ones constructed for this study, but accounting for wealth as well. Analyses with such indicators may help explain, for example, why the 70+ age group in Table 1 shows the least difference across SES indicators. While currently there are no coherent national datasets in Australia that simultaneously contain variables on disability, family income, family size and family wealth at the level of the individual, some are expected in future.

Another future development of interest is the extension of this cross-sectional study to a longitudinal one analysing the impact of population ageing on the various SES measures used. Population ageing is expected to have a significant impact on age distributions within the individual-based SES quintiles, but not within the SEIFA-based quintiles (Figure 8). For example, if present income-patterns by age remained unchanged over time then, as the population ages, the lower individual-based SES quintiles would contain a higher proportion of 70+ year olds - and thus higher disability rates - than currently. Thus, population ageing is expected to lead to a widening of health inequalities when using individual-based SES indicators – but to remain virtually unchanged with the geographic-area-based measures.

5.8 Choosing the SES indicators for DYNAMOD

In view of the conclusions reached in section 5.7, the individual-based indicators are to be preferred when estimating disability rates by SES. Because we used the 1998 Disability survey for estimating disability rates in this thesis, we could choose between the SEIFA and the individual indicators - since both types were available from that survey (section 5.2).

We chose the individual-level SES indicators for:

- imputing disability status by SES to persons in the model's Base data (Block 1 in Figure 1, section 1.5.1); and

- establishing changes in disability status by SES in the projection years (ie in the 'Simulation phase', Block 4 in Figure 1).[21]

The specification of the SES indicators in the above two instances, and their implementation in DYNAMOD, are described in Chapter 7.

---

[21] In that case the SEIFA was not an option because DYNAMOD has no geographic dimension.

78

However, when preparing the linked mortality and disability input data by SES (Block 2 in Figure 1), the situation became complicated by the fact that, for mortality, only the SEIFA indicator was available.

The question thus arose as to whether in this case it was preferable to choose the SEIFA index for estimating both the disability and mortality rates. The alternative was to use the SEIFA when estimating death rates, and an individual-based SES indicator when estimating disability rates. Because this latter option would have led to data-based inconsistencies in the variables and parameters estimated through the mathematical equations linking mortality and disability in the model (section 4.4), we chose the former option - that is use of the SEIFA as indicator of SES for both mortality and disability when preparing the Block 2 (Figure 1) input data. Chapter 6 describes how these input data were computed.

As the above indicates, due to only SEIFA-based indexes being available for mortality, we ended up using the SEIFA in the mortality-disability equations. For the simulation phase, only the family income-based indicators were available (because DYNAMOD has no geographic dimension). Thus, transitions in disability status were estimated using income-based SES indicators. The implications of this can be seen from the Table 2 findings. These indicate that, compared with the income-based indicators, the SEIFA underestimates differences in disability rates between low and high SES groups. As a result, inequalities in the mortality rates predicted by the model will be somewhat lesser than inequalities predicted in disability rates.

Chapter 6   Preparing the input data on mortality and disability by age, sex and socioeconomic status

The research reported in this Chapter concerns the mortality and disability related input data required for implementation of the Health_SES module – see block 2 in Figure 1 (section 1.5.1). It is published in Walker (2002). As indicated in Chapter 3, the data sources used were an extract from the AIHW's Mortality database (1995-97) and the ABS's 1998 Disability survey. The input data EXCEL sheets are available to examiners on request. Chapter 4 described the way these input data are made use of in the model.

6.1 Introduction

The mortality and disability input data needed for the model by sex, SEIFA quintiles and single years of age (0 to 104) – to assign values to the variables and parameters of the equations in section 4.4 – comprises the following elements:

- mortality rates – the probability of death for the able-bodied (who die from external causes), the disabled (who die from non-external causes), and the population in general (ie able-bodied plus disabled). In the model, the date of death is computed as a function of disability – that is, the disabled have lower life expectancies than the able bodied;

- mortality improvement rates, covering three periods: 1987 to 1994, 1995 to 2004 and 2005 to 2050 . These are based on ABS predictions and account for expected future increases in life expectancies;

- disability prevalences - computed by as the number disabled in each age-sex-SES cell divided by the total number of persons in that cell;

- disablement rate - a function of the number becoming disabled, the number of recoveries, the able-bodied population, and the number of deaths in the able bodied population; and

- recovery rate – as estimated using the equations of section 4.4.2.

Each of these elements of the input data set were computed outside the model, and prepared in the same format as for the original version of DYNAMOD. The effect of separately presenting information for 'five SES quintiles' – compared with 'all quintiles' previously – was that the new input dataset became five times longer than the original, with data set out sequentially from SES quintile 1 to SES quintile 5.

The way each of these elements were calculated using the relevant data sources is described below (sections 6.2 to 6.4).

6.2   *Mortality rates*

6.2.1   *By SES quintiles*

To compute separate mortality rates for the able-bodied and disabled populations by SEIFA quintiles, we used the first set of equations in section 4.4. It was possible to obtain such separate mortality rates by using data from two sources: the AIHW extract for mortality by age, sex and SES, and the 1998 Disability Survey for disability prevalence by SES. This was because – as the equations indicate - the disability prevalence rate mathematically links the able-bodied population to the disabled population.

Mortality rates were initially computed by sex, SEIFA quintile and 5-year age groups and then smoothed – using the GAM spline program of SAS[22] – to produce rates for single years of age.

As an example of the results obtained by SES, Figure 9 presents mortality rates for males from external causes (such as accidents and suicides). As expected, the Figure shows that males aged 15-39 years had exceptionally high such mortality rates (compared with most older age groups). The Figure also shows that quintile 1 people consistently had the highest mortality rates, and quintile 5 the lowest - with quintiles 2, 3 and 4 falling in between.

Figure 9: **Mortality rates, external causes, males age, SEIFA quintiles, 1995-7**

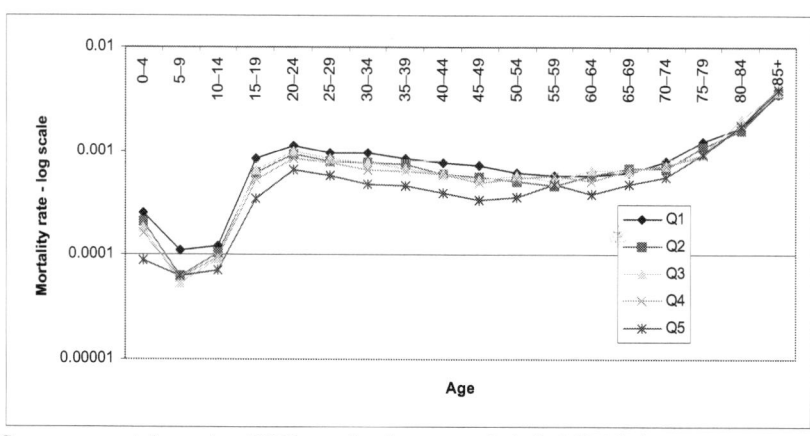

Sources: computations using AIHW mortality data extract. Quintile 1 (Q1) is the most disadvantaged and Q5 the least disadvantaged.

---

[22] The GAM procedure of SAS fits generalised additive models, based on nonparametric regression and smoothing techniques. Nonparametric regression relaxes the usual assumption of linearity. The GAM procedure combines the additivity assumption (which enables nonparametric relationships to be explored simultaneously) with the distributional flexibility of generalised linear models.

We found that this ranking remained consistent not only with all classes of mortality, but also across all the other aspects of the input data required by the model. This is remarkable, given that the various rates were computed using data from several unrelated sources, and were linked through complex equations (section 4.4). For all-cause mortality – Figure A4.3, Appendix A4 - we found the pattern to age 39 to be similar to that in Figure 9. However, for the over 40 age groups all cause mortality rates were found to be well above those in Figure 9.

Figure A4.3 also shows that differences in mortality rates across SEIFA quintiles were greater for men than women, and that - across all age groups - all cause mortality rates were higher for men than for women.

The above illustrates the dominance of illness-related deaths after age 40 and the much greater importance of 'external cause' related deaths for younger persons. The decision to model mortality from external and non-external causes separately was taken in response to these findings – see sections 3.4, 4.2.1 and 4.4.1.

6.2.2 Over time

Because in the simulation phase DYNAMOD projects life events into the future, there is a need to have trend information on mortality and disability rates – preferably from historical data. By comparing mortality statistics from the model's original 1990-92 input data (by age and sex) with the new 1995-97 data (by age, sex and SEIFA quintile), it was possible to examine how mortality rates changed between the early and mid 1990s. Figure 10 illustrates this for males, for non-external causes and - for sake of readability - for all SES quintiles. We chose non-external causes (ie the disabled), because for people dying from 'external' causes (ie the able-bodied) historical data suggested that mortality rates had changed very little over time.

83

Figure 10 shows that even in this relatively short five-year period, mortality rates from non-external causes declined significantly. This is consistent with the general trend towards increasing life expectancies.

Distinction between the sexes was also found to be important, since Figure A4.1 (Appendix A4) indicates that in both time periods, and for most age groups, all cause mortality rates were significantly lower for women than for men. Although not charted, the differences across SEIFA quintiles were also found to be significantly smaller for women than for men. Statistics for all cause mortality and for non-external causes (Figures A4.1 and A4.2) both indicate a decline in mortality rates in the 1995-97 period compared with the 1990-92 period - with the trend being considerably stronger for mortality arising from non-external causes.

Figure 10: **Mortality rates for men, non-external causes (ie the disabled population), by single years of age, 1990-92 and 1995-97**

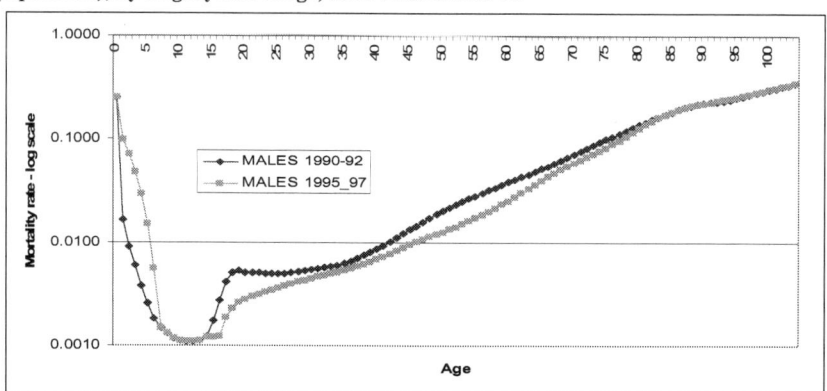

Sources: input data to DYNAMOD (ABS, 1993 (Walker and Abello, 2000, section 6.8) and computations for this thesis (AIHW extract, 1995-97).

6.3 Disability prevalence

A striking feature of Figure 11 - which plots the proportion disabled by single years of age for 1993 and for 1998 - is the steady and accelerating increase in disability rates from age 40 onwards. Appendix A5, Figure A5.1 - which shows these rates by sex - indicates that, by age 80, around 60% of men and 50% of women have become 'disabled'. Another noteworthy feature of Figure A5.1 is that the onset of disability occurs at younger ages for men than for women.

Unlike the trend for mortality (Figure 10), Figure 11 suggests that disability rates generally increased over time.

Figure 11: **Disability prevalence, males, by age, 1993 and 1998**

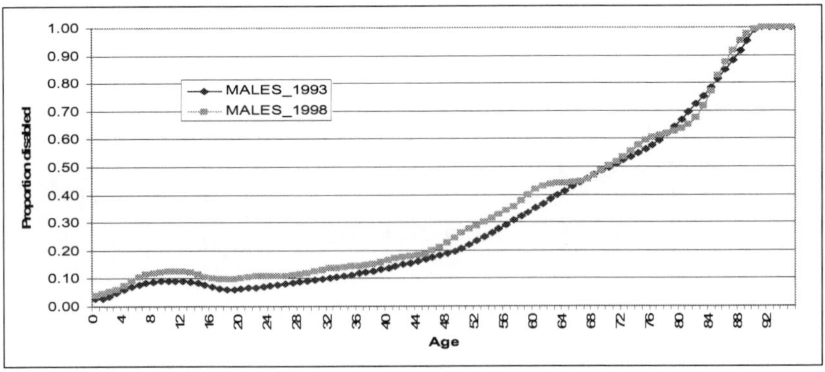

Sources: ABS Disability surveys (1993 and 1998). Note that in these surveys years of age above 85 are available as a single 85+ grouping.

Although this pattern may arise from differences in survey design across the 1993 and 1998 Disability surveys (section 9.2), earlier studies indicated a similar pattern using different data sources. For example, studying four National Health Surveys between 1983 and 1995, Walker and Abello (2000) observed steady increases in the number of Australians reporting serious illnesses, and in the number of doctor visits per person, per year. Amongst possible explanations for the apparent worsening of health on average put forward by these authors are that modern technology may keep the disabled alive longer and that - due to more frequent doctor visits - people are now aware of, and thus declare, a greater number of their illness-related disabilities than previously.

As for mortality rates, the disability data by SEIFA quintile indicated a consistently higher prevalence rate for quintile 1 people (the most disadvantaged) than for quintile 5 people. These findings are in line with those of earlier studies (Chapter 2).

6.4 Disability decrement rates

Disability decrement rates were derived using standard multiple decrement techniques (Antcliff et al, 1996). Briefly, the able bodied population is subject to exits due to death and disability and entrants due to recovery, while the disabled population is subject to exits due to death and recovery and entrants due to onset of disability.

We assumed that, for all SEIFA quintiles, the recovery patterns specified in the original input dataset – Antcliff et al (1996) - remained unchanged. For the new input data we then only needed to compute, by SEIFA quintile, the number - and rate - of people becoming disabled. We did this using equations 5, 6 and 7 in section 4.4. Our computed disablement rates for all quintiles were of the same order of magnitude as the rates originally specified for the model. As noted earlier, the input data EXCEL sheets are available to examiners on request.

Chapter 7   Modelling socioeconomic status for the Base dataset and the projection years

This Chapter reports on the development of more complex, individual level and income-based indicators of SES, than those generally used in the literature. In particular taking account of wealth in DYNAMOD's simulation phase, as well as the traditional income and family size variables, is an advance on traditional methods. This is because cash incomes do not reflect the total resources available to families. Since people generally accumulate wealth as they age, not accounting for wealth in indicators of SES will result in allocation of older people to lower SES quintiles than if wealth had also been accounted for (Chapter 5).

The sections below concern Blocks 1 and 4 in Figure 1 (section 1.5.1).

7.1 Modelling socioeconomic status in the Base dataset

To impute to the Base dataset the income and wealth-based SES indicators used in the simulation phase (section 7.2) first constructed an indicator using two variables already in that dataset: total income and superannuation (the only indicator of wealth in that dataset (section 1.4 and section A1.2 of Appendix A1), as wealth only starts being accumulated in the simulation years). To obtain in each simulation year a consistent indicator of socioeconomic status, we added a family's *annual* income to the *annual* equivalent of the family's total superannuation in that year (section A1.2, Appendix A1). To convert total superannuation into an annuity[23] we used a constant, 0.052 - the observed 5.2% rate of return on renting private dwellings in 1998. This reflects the fact that most of the wealth of Australians arises from home ownership (Kelly et al 2004).

---

[23] The method used is similar to that adopted by the ABS when estimating annual service flow figures from fixed capital stock data (ABS 2000c, Chapter 11, paragraphs 11.32 to 11.38).

SES status in the Base dataset is thus given by:

SES_status = yearly income + annualised superannuation

Next we summed individuals' SES_status within each family and allocated that summed value to each family member. Finally, we sorted the Base population by their families' SES_status and divided the total population into five equal parts – thus creating the variable 'SES quintile', each quintile accounting for 20% of the total population.

In the Base dataset there was also a need to re-impute disability status to each individual. This was because in the original Base dataset disability was only allocated by age and sex and we now required an allocation by SES as well. As the basis for this imputation we constructed a family income[24] variable from the ABS's 1998 Disability survey. We also incorporated a scaling factor, which was chosen so that the distribution of disability in the model's output for 1998 - by age, sex and SES - closely matched the same distribution in the 1998 Disability survey.

7.2 Modelling socioeconomic status in the simulation years

Due to the wide range of variables available in DYNAMOD, we were able to construct SES indicators for its simulation phase that better reflected the economic resources available to families (section 5.2) than in other parts of the model. Apart from income (earned and government cash benefits) and family size, DYNAMOD has an indicator of family wealth that is accumulated over people's lives (Kelly 2002; 2003). Income is important because, out of the indicators of SES used in the literature, family income is considered to be the single most effective summary measure of SES (Vinson 1999).

---

[24] A family income-based indicator was the closest to the SES indicator in the Base data, since the Disability survey has no information on superannuation or wealth.

However, Headey and Wooden (2004) noted that income was an imperfect measure of the economic circumstances of households, and demonstrated that wealth - which can be viewed as providing a degree of economic security - was at least as important as income.

Because people tend to accumulate wealth as they age, their SES may not decline in line with their cash incomes once they leave the workforce. Thus, data permitting, wealth should be accounted for in measures of SES. Finally, as shown in section 5.2, family size is also important, and we accounted for this once again using the modified OECD scale factor (Appendix A8).

Based on the above, a preferred SES measure would be one that was a function of yearly 'equivalent family income' as well as an annualised indicator of wealth.

Three different SES indicators were constructed within the simulation phase of the model, each computed in DYNAMOD at the end of the relevant financial year:

Income = Family income (earned + government benefits);

Income_Wealth = Family income (earned + government benefits) + annualised wealth[25]

Equivalent Income_Wealth = {family income (earned+government benefits) + annualised family wealth} / equivalence scale factor.

The Income indicator was chosen because it is often used in the literature (usually in cases where no other data are available). Next the Income_Wealth indicator was simulated, followed by the Equivalent Income_Wealth measure – thus building up to the indicator that was shown above to best reflect the economic resources available to

[25] To convert wealth into an annuity we used the same constant, 0.052, as for annualised super in the Base data (section 7.1). The method used is similar to that adopted by the ABS when estimating annual service flow figures from fixed capital stock data (ABS 2000c, Chapter 11, paragraphs 11.32 to 11.38).

families. Equivalent income indicators are also the most commonly used SES measures in socioeconomic studies[26] - with equivalent income deciles being often available in ABS statistical collections - ABS (2003a and b).

Examining in Chapter 5 the reasons why inequality estimates – that is differences between the disability rates of the rich and the poor – differed between types of individual-based SES indicators we found that, as the definition of the SES indicator changed, the allocation of persons of a given age and health status to an SES quintile also changed (Figure 8). This means, for example, that choosing the Income_Wealth indicator in DYNAMOD will lead to more older persons being allocated to SES quintile 3 (and less to SES quintile 2) than with the Income indicator. Accounting for wealth as well as income will have the greatest impact on the allocation of the elderly, because people accumulate wealth as they age (section A1.2, Appendix A1). Allocating more older persons to quintile 3 will in turn result in an increase in the proportions disabled in that quintile (and a decrease in quintile 2). A preliminary investigation of these issues can be found in Walker (2003).

---

[26] Without considering wealth, generally due to lack of suitable data.

Chapter 8   Modelling health state transitions

The key innovation in this Chapter is the building, into the enhanced model, the progression of chronic diseases – and thus disability - over the life courses of individuals. An important advance that this innovation results in is the ability to link health with a person's 'functionality' - which in turn can be linked to people's ability to remain in the labour force (Chapter 12) or to live independently. With such links between health and functionality, it becomes possible to study the financial consequences for individuals and for government of changes in people's health status (Chapters 11 and 12).

The key challenge in this Chapter was the lack of longitudinal data from which to estimate health state transitions. This was overcome through the development - for purposes of this thesis - of a methodology for estimating health state transitions from cross-sectional data.

The research described below concerns Blocks 1, 2 and 4 in Figure 1 (section 1.5.1). Because severity of chronic diseases – and the related disabilities – impact on quality of life, on health care costs and on the extent of financial support by the government to the disabled, we redefined the original (0,1) disability variable so that it now has four levels, progressing from no long-term illness to severe disability.

The sections below describe how 'health state transitions' were defined and incorporated into DYNAMOD, once it had the Health_SES module added to it.

8.1 The available data

In DYNAMOD changes in the status of individuals – such as their marital status - are usually determined either through hazard functions or transition probabilities. For modelling health state transitions, there are no Australian longitudinal data suitable for estimating hazard functions. We were thus constrained to use cross sectional data – which was available in the 1998 Disability survey (ABS 1999a, b, c).

In that survey disability is defined in terms of the restrictions it places on every day core activities (section 3.2). Each person is classified into one of eight health/disability classes (ABS 1999a): (1) 'has disability and is *profoundly* restricted in core activities'; (2) 'has disability and is *severely* restricted in core activities'; (3) 'has disability and is *moderately* restricted in core activities'; (4) 'has disability and is *mildly* restricted in core activities'; (5)'has disability and is *not restricted* in core activities but restricted in schooling or employment'; (6) 'has disability and is *not restricted* in core activities, schooling or employment'; (7) 'has a long-term health condition without disability'; (8) 'has no long-term health condition'.

Figure 12 presents the proportion of the population by age and health status in 1998 - with (1) and (2) grouped into a 'Disab_severe' class; (3) and (4) into a 'Disab_mild' class; and (5) and (6) into a 'Disab_no restriction' category. A striking feature of the Figure is the importance of age in determining the likelihood of being disabled. It shows that while the proportion disabled in 1998 was only around 20% up to age 30, that proportion increased to close to 50% by age 50 and reached 85-90% for ages 75 and over. Although based on cross sectional data, the Figure also suggests that people generally progressed, as they aged, from a state of no long-term illness to long-term illness, and then to progressively more restrictive forms of disability.

Figure 12: **Per cent of the population by age and health status, 1998**

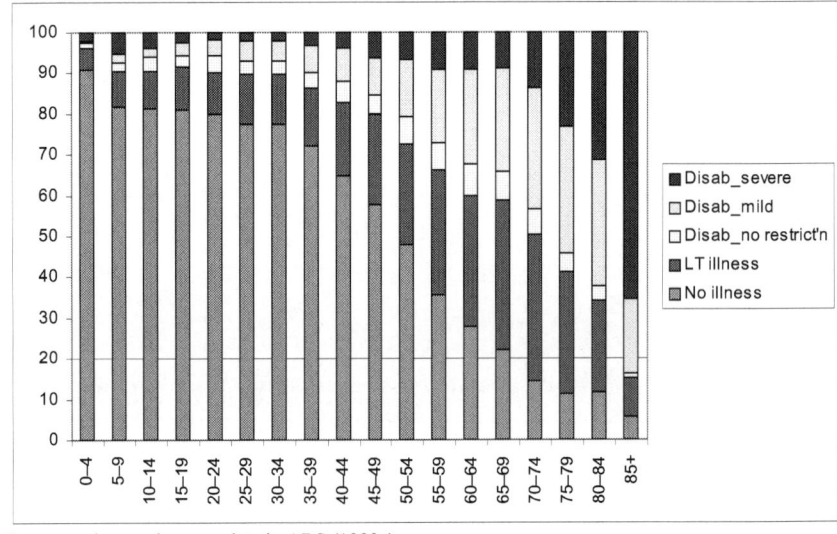

Source: unit record survey data in ABS (1999a)

Appendix A7 shows that the age by health-state patterns were found to be similar for men and women, although there were some differences. For example, up to age 40 a lower proportion of women had a severe disability than men (Figures A7.2.1 and A7.2.2). A possible reason for this is that women generally live longer – with life expectancies at birth in 2000 being 77 years for men and 82 years for women (Dunn et al, 2002).

The pattern was similar for mild disability, but generally a higher proportion of women had long term illnesses than men. With regard to 'no long term illness', a significantly higher proportion of women were disease or accident free up to the age of 25, but beyond that age there did not seem to be much difference between the sexes (section A7.2).

8.2   The health states modelled

To make the modelling task manageable, we reduced the eight health classes in the 1998 Disability survey (section 8.1 and section A2.3, Appendix A2) to four health states:

1. 'No long-term illness' being: 'has no long-term health condition';

2. 'Long-term illness' being: 'has a long-term health condition' and/or disability with 'no impact on core activities';

3. 'Disab_mild' being: has disability with 'mild or moderate impact on core activities';

4. 'Disab_severe' being: has disability with 'severe or profound impact on core activities'.

8.3   Methodology for estimating health transition probabilities

To estimate health transition probabilities a new four-health-states variable was constructed – defined in section 8.2 – with the last two combined accounting for the disabled group.

8.3.1   Assumptions

Two assumptions needed to be made to enable transition probabilities to be estimated from cross-sectional data (ABS 1999a). The first was that age was the key driver of disability and its severity. Evidence for this was presented in section 8.1 (Figure 12). The second assumption was that health states always progressed from a particular health state to a worse one – that is that 'recovery' was not possible.

94

While this assumption is clearly not always correct, 'recovery' at the age groups and the

levels of aggregations we are mainly concerned with was shown by the available data to

be a rare event.[27] Also, steady progression from mild versions of a disease to more

severe forms, as people with chronic diseases age, has been demonstrated by the

longitudinal data available in some developed countries (such as the extensive

longitudinal data on diabetes at the Diabetes Trial Unit, Oxford University, UK).

For the simulation phase the 'steady-state assumption' – defined in section 2.6 - was

adopted re the health transition probabilities. This assumption, seen as useful as a

benchmark in the development phase (Spielaue 2002), can be relaxed in the later stages

of development, with the probabilities changing over time in line with expected future

trends.

8.3.2 Computing health transition probabilities

The four health states were disaggregated by age groups: 0-14, 15-24, 25-44; 45-54; 55-

64; 65-69; 70-74 and 75 or above (8 classes);[28] by sex (2 classes); and by quintiles of

family-income-based socioeconomic status (5 classes).[29] These levels of disaggregation

meant that transition probabilities had to be estimated for 8*5*2=80 groupings (or

cells).

Table 4 presents the matrix equations for estimating transition probabilities in general.

---

[27] Note that with the (0,1) disability variable, 'recovery' is modelled in the original version of DYNAMOD. The input data assembled for that version shows that 'recovery' mainly occurs in younger age groups for conditions such as injuries and asthma, and is very rare for older people with chronic diseases.

[28] The age groups were selected so that they matched the groups used in DYNAMOD's Labour force Module (ie 15-24, 25-44 and 45+); that they covered all ages (so we added the 0-14 group); and that they were more disaggregated the older people were (since severity of disability increased considerably in older age groups).

[29] Which of the three SES indicators available in the simulation phase is closest to the SEIFA (used for mortality) could not be assessed because (a) DYNAMOD does not have a geographic dimension, and (b) the Disability survey – which is the source of both the SEIFA and the family income indicators - does not have data on wealth.

Table 4: Matrix algebra equations for transition probabilities - general notation

$$
\begin{bmatrix}
P[D_{0(a+1)}] \\
P[D_{1(a+1)}] \\
P[D_{2(a+1)}] \\
P[D_{3(a+1)}]
\end{bmatrix}
=
\begin{bmatrix}
P[D_{0(a+1)}|D_{0(a)}] & P[D_{0(a+1)}|D_{1(a)}] & P[D_{0(a+1)}|D_{2(a)}] & P[D_{0(a+1)}|D_{3(a)}] \\
P[D_{1(a+1)}|D_{0(a)}] & P[D_{1(a+1)}|D_{1(a)}] & P[D_{1(a+1)}|D_{2(a)}] & P[D_{1(a+1)}|D_{3(a)}] \\
P[D_{2(a+1)}|D_{0(a)}] & P[D_{2(a+1)}|D_{1(a)}] & P[D_{2(a+1)}|D_{2(a)}] & P[D_{2(a+1)}|D_{3(a)}] \\
P[D_{3(a+1)}|D_{0(a)}] & P[D_{3(a+5)}|D_{1(a)}] & P[D_{3(a+1)}|D_{2(a)}] & P[D_{3(a+1)}|D_{3(a)}]
\end{bmatrix}
\begin{bmatrix}
P[D_{0(a)}] \\
P[D_{1(a)}] \\
P[D_{2(a)}] \\
P[D_{3(a)}]
\end{bmatrix}
$$

Table 5: Matrix algebra equations for transition probabilities - assuming that people's health can only deteriorate

$$
\begin{bmatrix}
P[D_{0(a+1)}] \\
P[D_{1(a+1)}] \\
P[D_{2(a+1)}] \\
P[D_{3(a+1)}]
\end{bmatrix}
=
\begin{bmatrix}
P[D_{0(a+1)}|D_{0(a)}] & 0 & 0 & 0 \\
P[D_{1(a+1)}|D_{0(a)}] & P[D_{1(a+1)}|D_{1(a)}] & 0 & 0 \\
P[D_{2(a+1)}|D_{0(a)}] & P[D_{2(a+1)}|D_{1(a)}] & P[D_{2(a+1)}|D_{2(a)}] & 0 \\
P[D_{3(a+1)}|D_{0(a)}] & P[D_{3(a+1)}|D_{1(a)}] & P[D_{3(a+1)}|D_{2(a)}] & P[D_{3(a+1)}|D_{3(a)}]
\end{bmatrix}
\begin{bmatrix}
P[D_{0(a)}] \\
P[D_{1(a)}] \\
P[D_{2(a)}] \\
P[D_{3(a)}]
\end{bmatrix}
$$

There is a set of equations of that type for each particular data 'cell', out of the total of 80 cells. To make the text easier to understand, an example 'cell' was chosen - Males in Quintile 1 moving from the 45-54 age group to the 55-64 age group.

Let: - $P[D_{0(a)}]$ be the probability that a 45-54 yo Male is in the 'No illness' category, with subscripts 1, 2 and 3 (instead of '0') referring to the 'Long-term illness' and the mild/severe disabled categories

- $P[D_{0(a+1)}|D_{0(a)}]$ indicate the conditional probability that, when that man in the 'No illness' class progresses to the next age group, he will remain in the 'No illness' class

- $P[D_{1(a+1)}|D_{0(a)}]$ indicate the conditional probability that, when that man progresses to the next age group, he will move to the 'Long-term illness' class, etc.

The assumption that people's health state can only get worse (section 8.3.1) led to many of the conditional probabilities being zeros. This is illustrated in Table 5 (presented below Table 4).

Using data from the 1998 Disability survey, we were able to estimate the probabilities in the first and the last columns of the Table 4 equations. To estimate the conditional probabilities in the middle columns, we first used the multiplication theorem of matrix algebra and then assigned plausible values to these probabilities ensuring that they were consistent with the 1998 Disability survey data.

The matrix algebra equations are:

$$P[D_{0(a+1)}] \ = \ P[D_{0(a+1)}|D_{0(a)}] * P[D_{0(a)}] \tag{1}$$

which can be solved uniquely for the conditional probability $P[D_{0(a+1)}|D_{0(a)}]$

$$P[D_{1(a+1)}] \ = \ P[D_{1(a+1)}|D_{0(a)}] * P[D_{0(a)}] + P[D_{1(a+1)}|D_{1(a)}] * P[D_{1(a)}] \tag{2}$$

$$P[D_{2(a+1)}] \ = \ P[D_{2(a+1)}|D_{0(a)}] * P[D_{0(a)}] + P[D_{2(a+1)}|D_{1(a)}] * P[D_{1(a)}] +$$
$$P[D_{2(a+1)}|D_{2(a)}] * P[D_{2(a)}] \tag{3}$$

$$P[D_{3(a+1)}] = P[D_{3(a+1)}|D_{0(a)}] * P[D_{0(a)}] + P[D_{3(a+1)}|D_{1(a)}] * P[D_{1(a)}] +$$

$$P[D_{3(a+1)}|D_{2(a)}] * P[D_{2(a)}] + P[D_{3(a+1)}|D_{3(a)}] * P[D_{3(a)}] \qquad (4)$$

The non-zero transitional probability values - obtained partly through equations (1) to (4) – were estimated so that the transition probabilities for each 'transition' column summed to 1.00. Results for the example 'cell' are in Table 6.

Table 6: **Example of a transition probability matrix: Quintile 1 Males moving from the 45-54 age group to the 55-64 age group**

	55_64 yo			$D_{0(a)}$	$D_{1(a)}$	$D_{2(a)}$	$D_{3(a)}$	45-54 yo
No illness	0.201	0.201		0.634	0.000	0.000	0.000	0.317
LT illness	0.310	0.310		0.327	0.950	0.000	0.000	0.218
Mild disab	0.309	0.309		0.030	0.030	0.980	0.000	0.299
Severe disab	0.180	0.180		0.009	0.020	0.020	1.000	0.167
Sum	1.000	1.000		1.000	1.000	1.000	1.000	1.000

The first and last columns contain accurately estimated probabilities for 55-64 and 45-54 year olds (ie population proportions from the 1998 Disability survey). The shaded column contains the 'matrix algebra' products based on the 45-54 age group's actual probabilities. We assigned values to the non-zero conditional probabilities so that their 'matrix algebra' product with the 45-54 age group's probabilities amounted to a value close to the known 55-64 probabilities.[30]

---

[30] While close to exact matches were obtained for most of the tables, in some instances this was not possible. This occurred in particular in the younger age groups – eg due to children outgrowing disabilities such as those due to asthma. Also, because the survey data for quintile 5 proved unreliable, in the input data to DYNAMOD we used the quintile 4 transition matrix for quintile 5 persons as well.

8.4 Implementation in the model

8.4.1 Input data

An additional input dataset was prepared containing the transition probabilities from the 80 tables (in line with the example in Table 6). The input data EXCEL sheets are available to examiners on request.

8.4.2 Implementation in the Base dataset

We needed to impute health states from the 1998 Disability survey (ABS 1999a) to individuals in the Base dataset by age, sex and SES. This provided each person with a starting health status. New-born babies and immigrants entering Australia were allocated an initial health status of 'No illness or disability'.

8.4.3 Implementation in the simulation phase of the model

In each simulation year DYNAMOD was re-programmed to assess, using Monte Carlo methods, whether the health state of each person entering the next age group would change or not.

Using the example in section 8.3.2 (Table 6), and the related cumulative probabilities, a man without illness who just reached age 55 would be studied in DYNAMOD by comparing a (0 to 1) random number to the cumulative probabilities specified in the input data. Thus, if the random number fell below 0.634, then there would be no change in that man's health state. If however it fell between 0.634 and 0.961 (that is 0.634 + 0.327) then there would be a change in his health state to having at least one long-term illness – and so on.

Chapter 9   Validation

In the context of dynamic microsimulation Caldwell and Morrison (2000) defined validation as: "a proactive, diagnostic effort to ensure that the model's results are reasonable and credible." For such models validation is particularly important since potential users will need to be convinced that the myriads of individual or family-based 'decisions' modelled make sense at the aggregate level. That is, when taken together, the effects of all the varied individual decisions should match benchmark statistics on year-by-year changes in such variables as population, educational and employment structures, families' incomes and wealth, and individuals' health.

As with most modelling exercises, it would be unrealistic to expect a perfect match against all the benchmark statistics. The extent of the match that is acceptable is a matter of judgement - often constrained by limitations on the available resources or time. A useful practical guide is that, if a particular distribution – such as disability rates by age group – is too far from the benchmark, then the researcher may have failed to capture what in reality was the major contributing factor to the observed statistics.

Morrison (1999) states that a fundamental test of policy models rests with the quality of their outputs and their utility to users. Users will want to know how credible are the model's outputs, that is:

- how close to reality are its databases and the functions determining life course events; and

- how its aggregate outputs compare with published statistics.

It was in response to the first of the above points that DYNAMOD's Base data was originally developed using high quality official statistics – rather than using synthetically generated person records (section 2.6). This philosophy was also adopted in this thesis (section 1.4).

The text below presents comparisons of aggregate level outputs from DYNAMOD with the related published benchmark statistics. Validation is first presented for disability in the original model, followed by validation of the new modules added to DYNAMOD as part of this thesis.

9.1   *Disability in the original model*

Earlier researches described the calibration processes of the original version of the dynamic microsimulation model (section 1.4, footnote 4). This version relied on disability statistics from the 1993 Disability Survey, and on mortality data over the 1990-92 period.

As a first step in the validation process carried out for this thesis, we up-dated the calibration carried out by King et al (1999a, pp. 12-13) using 1998 data for disability and 1995-97 data for mortality. We then compared the up-dated results with those obtained with the early 1990s data. As a second step, the 1998 model outputs are validated against 1998 ABS benchmark statistics (section 9.2).

To do this, we extracted annual cross sectional snapshots for disability from the up-dated model's output. Using these data, age specific disability rates were computed for two of the simulation years, 1986 and 1998. These were selected because they allowed comparisons of the simulation results with the earlier validation exercise against the 1993 survey data. Disability rates per 1000 population were computed by age group, by first outputting the number of persons with a 'disabled' status, and next outputting the numbers in the total population.

Figure 13 charts the results for 1986 (the Base year), for 1998 (the year to which the enhanced version of the model has been re-based), and benchmark data from the 1993

Disability survey (which was used by earlier researchers for calibration purposes – see

King et al, 1999a, Figure 3).

Figure 13: **Age specific disability rates in the 1993 ABS survey and in DYNAMOD for 1986 and 1998**

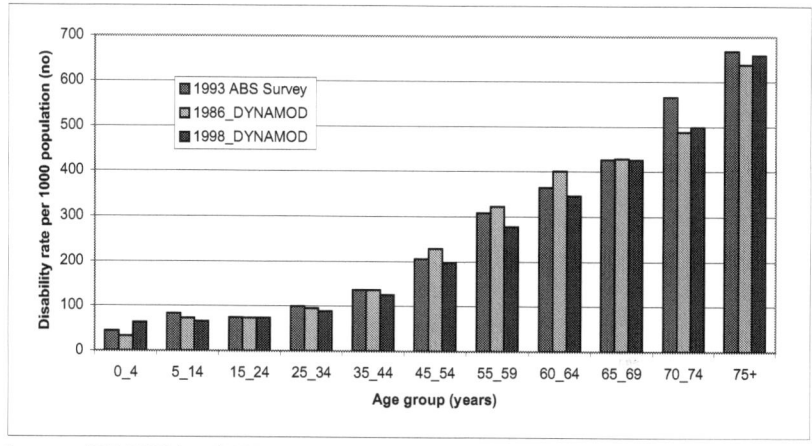

Sources: ABS (1993c) and DYNAMOD simulations.

As expected, for 1986 our results are very close to those reported by the earlier

validation team. Because of this our conclusion is in line with their observation that, for

1986, DYNAMOD appears "to underestimate the disability rates for the older age

groups" – King et al (1999a, p. 12). Overall, however, the patterns of age-specific

disability rates generated by DYNAMOD for 1986 and 1998 were both quite close to

the historical pattern obtained from the 1993 Disability survey.

9.2 Disability in the enhanced model

A common characteristic of all dynamic models is that their simulated outcomes do not

track comparable historical values with perfect accuracy. Caldwell (1996) confirmed

that, in this respect, dynamic microsimulation models are not different from other

models. Because such models are often developed to allow policy analyses to be carried

out with greater accuracy than with traditional methods, accurate tracking of historical benchmarks is crucial to their credibility. For that reason dynamic microsimulation models are often calibrated – or aligned – to published aggregate benchmark statistics (see 10.1.1).

In this section we describe the calibration of the new Health State Transition module, so that the cross-sectional disability patterns simulated for 1998 line up reasonably well with the official statistics in ABS (1999a). To carry out the calibration, the approach chosen was one in which interim outcomes from the simulation are used in the alignment procedure – the 'simulation alignment' approach described in Bækgaard 2002a. The approach can be implemented either by changing function parameters to produce an aligned outcome - called *parameter alignment* - or by adjusting the raw output from the model to produce aligned outcomes – called *ex-post alignment*. To calibrate the Health State Transition module we used the *ex-post alignment* procedure. For a discussion on the limitations of the approach see section 10.1.

Figure 14 compares the simulated distribution of the population in 1998 by health states with published ABS statistics. It shows that the calibration process achieved a good agreement.

Next, the transitions in the simulation phase of the model from one health state to the next were calibrated, so that changes over time in aggregate disability rates were broadly in line with historical trends. The four Disability surveys (1981, 1988, 1993 and 1998) indicated steadily *increasing* disability rates over time – from 14.6% in 1981 to 19.3% in 1998 (ABS 1999c, p. 19). This suggests a longer-term upward drift of 1.38% every five years. Across the last two surveys that increase was somewhat less: from a disability rate of 18.02% in 1993 to 19.3% in 1998 (or 1.28% over five years). For our study we needed to ascertain whether these trends were *(a)* 'real', or reflected to some extent a statistical artifice; and *(b)* were likely to continue in future.

Figure 14: **Proportion of disabled in the Australian population by health states, ABS survey and DYNAMOD, 1998**
(per cent)

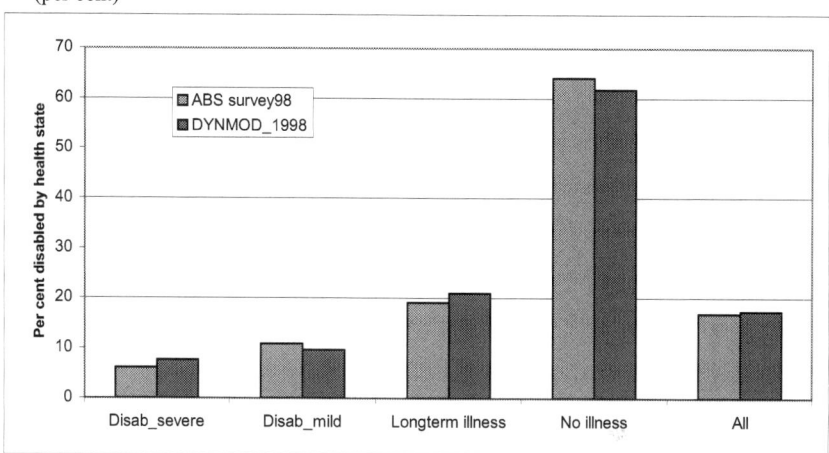

Sources: 1998 Disability survey (ABS 1999a) and simulations with DYNAMOD.

With respect to (a), the ABS reported that the greater part of the increase between 1993 and 1998 was for people with severe and profound restrictions (ABS 1999c, p.6). This suggests that improved medical technology may have had the effect of keeping disabled people alive longer. This is supported by the conclusion of Davis et al (2002, p.1) – gained through a study across four ABS Disability surveys – that two thirds or more of the increase in life expectancy over the decade 1988 to 1998 was taken in a state of disability. However, the Australian Institute of Health and Welfare (AIHW 2003a and 2001) noted that the rise in the overall number of people with disability between the 1993 and 1998 surveys – especially those with severe or profound core activity restrictions – was in large part due to changes in survey methods. Nevertheless the AIHW expected future disability rates to rise in the next 10 years as the baby boomers moved up the population pyramid.

The 2003 Disability survey - currently being processed by the ABS – maintains the methods used in the 1998 survey. Thus, once it becomes available, the direction and magnitude of trends in disability rates between 1998 and 2003 should be less confused.

With respect to (b), Manton and XiLiang (2001) found – based on the US '1999 National Long-Term Care Survey'– that disability rates amongst 65+ year olds in the United States actually declined between 1982 and 1999. In a similar vain, O'Connell (2003) reports on a UK longitudinal study which found that, between 1981 and 1995, there were fewer years in poor health than in good health for those aged 65 years or more.

For Australia, these international trends could possibly signal slower increases in disability rates in future, especially since the 2001 National Health Survey by the ABS indicates a slowing of the upward trend in the proportion of people with chronic diseases (and thus with related disabilities) -Walker et al (2003).

Based on the above, we calibrated DYNAMOD so that its simulated future disability rates increased at a considerably slower rate than was indicated by the 1993 and 1998 ABS Disability surveys. That is, the national disability rate in DYNAMOD's Base case – a 'past trends continue' simulation - increases by 0.43% every 5 years. This compares with 1.28% across the last two Disability surveys, with much of this arising from differences in survey methods according to the AIHW. Once the direction of likely future trends becomes clearer, the model could be re-calibrated accordingly.

Chapter 10   Limitations

Like all models, microsimulation models simplify reality. This is in part because the available data rarely captures all aspects of the real world, but mainly because of the time and resource constraints applying to model building. The areas that can be left outside the model, and the amount of effort to be expanded on particular aspects of the model, are decided by the analyst on the basis on the key policy issues that the model is expected to provide answers for. Also, models that project into the future, such as DYNAMOD, will have assumptions built into them about 'default' future trends which in some cases can be altered by the analyst. The simplifications and assumptions adopted will inevitably lead to limitations that need to be borne in mind when examining the outputs produced by the model.

Apart from their need for longitudinal data - which is much less likely to be available in Australia than in many other developed countries (section 2.6, and Chapter 3) - the major limitations of dynamic microsimulation models arise from the fact that the methods for building such models are still evolving (section 10.1). Limitations of the model outputs reported in Chapters 11 and 12 can also arise from existing techniques not having been applied - due to the time and resource constraints that generally apply to PhD theses (section 10.3).

10.1 Alignment procedures

As noted in Chapter 9, with dynamic microsimulation there is a need to ensure that the myriads of individual or family-based 'decisions' modelled make sense at the aggregate level. Thus, how well the model is aligned to historical data - or to expected future developments - will have a considerable impact on the credibility of the model results.

Also, once model development is sufficiently advanced for policy relevant applications to be carried out, the automation of the simultaneous alignment of all key variables becomes important. This is because policy relevant applications require quick response to evolving requests from clients for simulating a wide range of possible future scenarios. The experience with the DYNAMOD applications reported in this thesis suggests that the current alignment processes are likely to be too inflexible and too slow for client-driven policy relevant applications.

The development of methodologies for aligning dynamic microsimulation models does not as yet seems to be at the stage where such automated methods can be contemplated. For example, to date there is no commonly accepted theory or agreed practice on how alignment should be carried out.

Given this situation, our coverage of this topic is limited to: (i) a summary of the sparse research on alignment issues – some published and some currently being developed (section 10.1.1); (ii) a description of the alignment processes used in DYNAMOD (section 10.1.2); and (iii) an assessment of the extent to which the current state of alignment methodologies and practices may affect the credibility of model outputs (10.1.3).

10.1.1 Alignment procedures in the literature

Neufeld (2000) defines alignment as a procedure which aims to achieve a match between the *average* (non-aligned) probability of an event occurring within a dynamic microsimulation model – for a particular event applying to a specific set of individuals in a given simulation year - and a related exogenously specified probability. In the case of DYNAMOD, the exogenously specified constraint is usually an aggregate statistic published by the ABS for event flows, such as birth or disability rates. For example, as will be seen in section 10.1.2, fertility rates in the original model were aligned to ABS benchmark statistics on actual and projected fertility rates.

Morrison (2001) describes the current status of alignment practices as follows:

"Most major longitudinal dynamic microsimulation models use some form of alignment. They commonly adjust econometrically estimated event probabilities to ensure that the expected proportions of events will reflect their desired assumptions or constraints. Increasingly, these models also employ alignment technologies to implement variance reduction, ensuring that the actual proportions of events conform closely to the assumed target proportions. Over time and across models, modellers have used a variety of techniques to adjust event probabilities and to choose the particular sets of events to be implemented. Gradually, the methods, formulae and algorithms have become more sophisticated. Successive enhancements have provided remedies for various shortcomings identified with earlier methods."

However, there is no commonly accepted theory regarding how alignment should be carried out."

In addition to there being no accepted theory, it is generally recognised that alignment of dynamic microsimulation models to actual data is difficult (Abello et al 2002). An example of relevance to this thesis is that, when aligning data on the proportion of people in four health states used in the Health State Transition module (Chapter 8), an improvement obtained in the alignment of the proportions in each health state by age group is likely to result in a worsening of the alignment obtained with other variables - ie by sex or SES or both. Ideally, alignment of the many life events – births, deaths, couple formation, disability, health, education, work, earnings, wealth, government benefits, etc – should be such that the best possible match to the combined set of all the official benchmark statistics is achieved.

Currently a group of model developers and users – associated with CORSIM, DYNACAN and PENSIM2 – has started to develop a theory able to guide the choice of alignment algorithms that could be generally accepted as 'best practice'. Research to date is still preliminary, with no official publications. Unpublished material includes a paper by Johnson (2001), which sets out what is meant by alignment and variance reduction; and what criteria are useful for comparing the effectiveness of various alignment methods. It then proceeds to applying such criteria to 'alignment by sorting' -

a particular technique that combines both alignment and variance reduction. In another unpublished document, Morrison (2001) makes contributions to both the theoretical and practical sides of the issue of alignment. On the theoretical side, this author develops a set of requirements or constraints that any alignment-variance-reduction method should meet. On the practical side, he proposes a particular method for determining appropriate probabilities. In a later note O'Donoghue (2003) studies the types of outputs produced by microsimulation models that in turn act as inputs into the alignment process - eg alignment as decision rules for discrete choice models determining such events as mortality, employment and disability; alignment for variables which are not estimated through equations in the model; alignment groups for transitions, durations, rates or totals; macro alignment; and alignment when behavioural change occurs. O'Donoghue then notes that the next steps will involve comparisons of the various alignment methods used in dynamic microsimulation models to date - for example the different methods for discrete choice models; methods for aligning distributions; the CORSIM_DYNACAN 'double pass' alignment method; and use of log linear models as an "alignment storage mechanism".

10.1.2 Alignment processes used in DYNAMOD

Because DYNAMOD took many years to develop, the issue of alignment only became important once the model started to produce simulation results. While in some cases the outputs produced by the model without alignment lined up well with benchmark statistics,[31] in others they diverged considerably from historical data.

As an example, the outputs produced by the non-aligned fertility module diverged substantially from benchmark statistics. Because of this, the fertility module had a complex alignment procedure added to it (Abello et al, 2002). Addition of the new

---

[31] Such as declines in mortality rates arising from increases in life expectancies. These were benchmarked to the related ABS projections.

109

alignment procedure resulted in a much improved match with benchmark data - Figure 15.

Details of the alignment processes used in the original version of DYNAMOD can be found in the model's documentation, listed in footnote 4, section 1.4. Those related to the modules added for purposes of this thesis are described in Chapter 9.

Figure 15: **Age-specific fertility rates: simulated average for 1994 to 1998 and ABS actual figures for 1996**

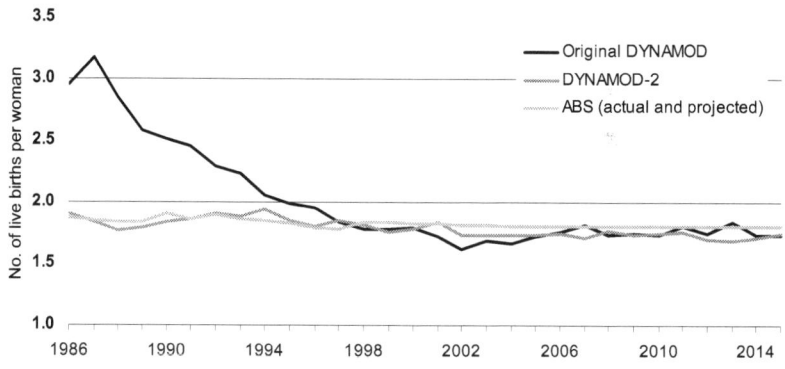

Source: Abello et al (2002, p.11).

10.1.3 Conclusion

At this time the lack of generally accepted 'best practice' methodologies for aligning dynamic microsimulation models is a major limitation. This arises partly because analysts have no way of knowing how close the alignment process is to an 'optimum' and, in the case of DYNAMOD, partly because its current alignment processes tend to be too inflexible and too slow for client-driven policy relevant applications. Another limitation is that, with current practices, analysts are unable to assess the variations in model outputs that would occur had a different alignment method been used.

Improvements in methodology may be possible in future, arising from research currently being carried out on alignment procedures (section 10.1.1).

10.2 Stochastic variations in model outputs

Abello et al (2002, p.30) note that, because in general human behaviour cannot be predicted, it is desirable for models like DYNAMOD to contain a random or stochastic element. As many functions in the model include at least one random element, it is likely that without alignment no two runs of the model would produce the same results (section 1.4).

Abello et al (2002, section 7.2) studied stochastic variation with the earlier, non-aligned version of DYNAMOD. These authors examined variations in model outputs with regard to random number variation in the modules on mortality and disability. The study was carried out on three cohorts of individuals in the Base dataset, aged 0–4 years, 20–24 years and 40–44 years. The model was run 20 times over a 50-year period, and counts were made of the surviving population in the years 1996, 2006, 2016, 2026 and 2036.

Important conclusions were that:

- the extent of stochastic variation was slight - four runs providing a good indication of the mean result in the example studied;

- the extent of variation had far more to do with the risk of an event occurring and population size than with the length of the model run; and

- after 20 years, deviations for the populations of the three cohorts were less than 0.5% either side of the mean, and after 50 years they rose to around 5%.

Similar findings emerged from overseas studies. For example, Pudney and Sutherland (1993 and 1994) found, using a static tax-benefit microsimulation model for the UK, that replicating the results four times – compared with a single simulation - had a surprisingly small effect, resulting in a decrease in the width of confidence intervals by 12% or less.

Variations are expected to be even less with the aligned version of the DYNAMOD, due to the constraints imposed by the alignment process on model outputs. When running simulations for this thesis with the aligned version of the enhanced model, we noted that stochastic variation was virtually non-existent – with very close results obtained even across two runs.

For this reason, we did not study stochastic variation further.

10.3 Sensitivity testing

Because each simulation run is an experiment that generates a single numerical solution based on a particular set of model specifications, researchers often use sensitivity analysis to compute upper and lower bounds to the most likely set of model outputs - Zaidi and Rake (2001).

Due in part to the limited scope of the thesis, and in part to the illustrative nature of the applications in Chapters 11 and 12 (section 1.1.2) we did not carry out 'sensitivity testing' for this project. If in future such tests are contemplated, then preliminary experiments suggest that different assumptions about the 'upward drift' in disability prevalence rates should be one of the key areas for a sensitivity test. This is because a small change in the 'drift rate' was found to result in considerable changes in model outputs. Since for this thesis we chose a relatively low 'drift rate' based on other countries' statistics (section 9.2), a particularly relevant sensitivity test would be one with a higher 'drift rate'. Compared with the model outcomes under such a test, the results reported in this thesis are likely to appear to be underestimates of disability rates

– and the related 'life years lost' and health expenditures.

10.4 Multiple-module validation

Zaidi and Rake (2001) note that, where models are constructed from sub-modules, there

will be multiple sources of error and many levels at which validation can occur.

Although multiple-module validation is rarely used, it can offer additional insights into

the working of a microsimulation model. Caldwell (1996, p. 515) puts this issue as

follows:

"When the interaction among modules produces additional information on sources of error in
the overall model, the benefit for the analyst is additional leverage with which to improve the
model as a whole, as well as its individual components."

Based on the above, once DYNAMOD is sufficiently developed for client-driven

policy relevant applications to be carried out, consideration could be given to the

possibility of using multiple-module validation techniques.

PART 2: APPLICATIONS OF THE ENHANCED MODEL

In part 2 of the thesis two novel applications of the enhanced model are presented:

- the simulation of the health and financial impacts of a narrowing in health inequalities in Australia: the 'improved public health scenario' – Walker (2004a); and

- a study of the ability of older Australians to stay in the labour force, as their health deteriorates with age. The related simulations are carried out under a 'no policy change' scenario as well as the 'improved public health' scenario – Walker (2004b).

While these applications are highly policy relevant, the main reason for their inclusion in the thesis is to illustrate the type of applications that the enhanced model can usefully simulate.

Chapter 11   Narrower health inequalities

11.1 Description of scenario and assumptions

The first illustrative scenario evaluated in this thesis is one in which the health of all Australians is lifted to that of the most affluent 20% of the population (ie that of people in SES quintile 5). This group is generally seen as setting an upper bound for potential health improvements. Policies to bring this scenario about could involve early intervention programs for families at risk (section 2.7; McCain and Mustard 1999 and 2002), or the adoption of healthier lifestyles by lower SES groups – eg through own or government initiatives, or greater focus on prevention. Also, there is some evidence to suggest that reducing income inequality by raising the incomes of the poor improves their health and is likely to lead to narrower health inequalities (section 2.4).

Given the wide range of policies that could achieve this scenario's disability reductions, the cost estimates reported in this Chapter focus on the benefits of the scenario, without quantifying the cost of implementing the policies. The benefit estimates are, however, useful in indicating the order of magnitude of the intervention costs that would be worth considering - for example under a 'break-even' financial constraint.

For both the Base case and the scenario simulations, we chose the Income_Wealth measure as indicator of SES. We made this choice because it was shown to be the best indicator of resource use (section 7.2) and because it produced outputs that were most coherent with the SEIFA index used in the model's mortality and disability input datasets.

First, individuals' life courses are simulated between 1986 and 2018 for the Base case and the scenario, with results reported for 1998 – the year for which model results can be compared with official statistics – and a date 20 years later, that is 2018. Then results under the scenario are compared with those under the Base case.

To facilitate comparisons with earlier studies, we computed the deaths and numbers disabled that would occur in a particular year, had the scenario been implemented.

All the *assumptions* made in DYNAMOD as 'default' prior to adding the new modules apply to the simulations reported in this application. The main assumption of relevance to this Chapter is that the earned income and the government transfers that are projected into the future are in constant dollars, allowing for a 1 per cent per annum real growth in these variables. Wealth is then estimated in the model on the basis of variables such as household savings rates - with the simulated growth rates in wealth ending up being three to four times that of total incomes (Kelly 2002).

The key assumptions within the newly added modules are that the age, sex and SES specific mortality and disability rates embedded in the model's input dataset remain unchanged over the simulation period; and the nationwide disability rate rises by 0.43% per cent every 5 years (Chapters 8 and 9). As with most 'default' settings, these assumptions can be changed if required.

The simulations under the scenario assume that the lifting of the health of all Australians to that of the most affluent 20% of the population occurs 'instantaneously' in 1986 – the year when the simulation starts.

11.2 *Impact on the number of deaths*

The number of deaths simulated for 1998 and 2018 under the Base case and the scenario are presented in Table 7. For 1998 it is estimated that 8.0% of deaths (10,197) would not have occurred, had the scenario been implemented (13,682 in 2018). An earlier paper Walker (2004a) estimated 'years of lives saved' as 183,300 in 1998 and 185,000 in 2018, assuming that for all those whose death would be deferred under the scenario would live to age 75.

Because we assumed that the patterns of mortality (and disability) rates in 1998 – by age, sex and SES - remained unchanged throughout the simulation period, differences between the 1998 and 2018 results in Table 7 arise mainly from population growth and population ageing.

The negative mortality differences for children are counter-intuitive and arise mainly from model characteristics. First, because mortality rates amongst children are relatively low, the stochastic nature of the Monte Carlo allocation method (sections 1.4 and 10.2) can on occasions lead to negative values. Second, the mortality and disability input data did not, in all age-sex cells, show the progressive SES Q1 to Q5 changes apparent at the aggregate level. Third, the smoothing of the mortality and disability input data (sections 6.2 and 6.3) may have also affected the pattern of progression from Q1 to Q5 (eg may have produced higher infant/child mortality rate in the top quintile than in the other quintiles). In future applications it would be possible to correct for input-data-related negative values - unless the data was considered to be accurate at the level of these age-sex cells. Regarding the Monte Carlo-related negative values, either aggregating the earlier age groups, or only presenting results for the groups aged 15 years or over would be appropriate.

In the 75+ age group – the one in which close to 70% of all deaths occurred - the estimated difference in the number of deaths between the Base case and the scenario is very small. This is likely to be due, in part, to life expectancies converging on zero fairly rapidly over the age of 75 in all SES quintiles – a pattern embedded in the mortality input data.

Table 7: **Number of deaths by age, 1998 and 2018**

Age group	Base Case No of deaths a	Scenario No of deaths b	Differences in number of deaths* (a-b)	Per cent change in number of deaths* 100*(a-b)/a
	1998			%
0_4	1,854	2,369	-515	-27.8
5_14	721	1,030	-309	-42.9
15_24	1,442	1,133	309	21.4
25_34	2,163	1,545	618	28.6
35_44	2,678	1,133	1,545	57.7
45_54	2,575	1,339	1,236	48.0
55_64	6,180	3,811	2,369	38.3
65_74	28,325	24,411	3,914	13.8
75+	81,885	80,855	1,030	1.3
All	**127,823**	**117,626**	**10,197**	**8.0**
	2018			
0_4	1,648	721	927	56.3
5_14	412	515	-103	-25.0
15_24	1,030	927	103	10.0
25_34	1,751	927	824	47.1
35_44	2,369	1,133	1,236	52.2
45_54	3,708	1,442	2,266	61.1
55_64	9,579	7,210	2,369	24.7
65_74	38,316	32,754	5,562	14.5
75+	123,394	122,896	498	0.4
All	**182,207**	**168,525**	**13,682**	**7.5**

* These are deaths that would have been deferred had the scenario been implemented – that is if all Australians had the same mortality rate as people in the most affluent socioeconomic quintile.
Source: DYNAMOD simulations.

However, because mortality and disability are mathematically linked (section 4.4.2), part of the explanation will also be due to the SES-related differentials in disability prevalence rates. The very small differences in the incomes of most 65+ year olds (since some 70% have sufficiently low cash incomes to qualify for the age pension – section 3.2), as they impact on differences in disability rates, may provide another reason for the small mortality differences amongst 75+ year olds between the Base case and the scenario. Data that is better able to track income as it evolves over the life course – such as that collected in the Harvard Study of Adult Development (Vaillant 2002) – could

result in possibly greater, and more accurate estimates.[32]

11.3 Impact on numbers disabled and on health care and disability pension expenditures

Because health expenditure data recently became available by age groups (AIHW

2004), and because the prevalence and severity of disability are strongly related to age,

in this section we report on disability and the related health costs by age – using the

same age groups as in AIHW (2004).

11.3.1 Numbers disabled

Disability rates in Australia were estimated to be significantly lower under the scenario

than under the Base case - Table 8.

Had the scenario been implemented, there would have been 430,231 less disabled

Australians in 1998 and 468,135 less in 2018. Most of the gains would have occurred

amongst people aged 45 years or more.

Figure 16 shows that the proportion disabled is considerably lower under the scenario

than under the Base case. Figure 17, which charts these results by health state shows

that, while the overall pattern did not change markedly across the different simulations,

the proportion disabled under the scenario was somewhat lower than under the Base

case, and the proportion with 'no illness' was somewhat higher under the scenario.

---

[32] This US study, covering an over 50 year-long period, investigated whether the factors
leading to poor life adjustment in young adulthood – ie SES, marital discord, low level of
education of parents, etc – also 'doomed youth to a miserable old age' (Vaillant 2002, p.6).

Table 8: **Number of disabled by age, 1998 and 2018**

Age group	Base Case No disabled a	Scenario No disabled b	Difference in number disabled (a-b)	Per cent change in number disabled (a-b)/a
		1998		%
0_4	57,989	29,973	28,016	48.3
5_14	147,908	118,347	29,561	20.0
15_24	327,128	301,481	25,647	7.8
25_34	527,669	510,880	16,789	3.2
35_44	356,998	337,943	19,055	5.3
45_54	446,402	314,253	132,149	29.6
55_64	387,898	264,298	123,600	31.9
65_74	459,792	433,630	26,162	5.7
75+	536,424	525,712	10,712	2.0
All	**3,248,208**	**2,817,977**	**430,231**	**13.2**
		2018		
0_4	60,564	38,213	22,351	36.9
5_14	113,300	68,804	44,496	39.3
15_24	155,633	84,769	70,864	45.5
25_34	403,966	357,616	46,350	11.5
35_44	472,770	482,967	- 10,197	-2.2
45_54	700,297	553,522	146,775	21.0
55_64	667,440	490,795	176,645	26.5
65_74	719,867	676,607	43,260	6.0
75+	902,177	881,062	21,115	2.3
All	**4,196,014**	**3,727,879**	**468,135**	**11.2**

Source: DYNAMOD simulations.

Figure 16: **Proportion disabled in the population, Base case and Scenario, 1998 and 2018**

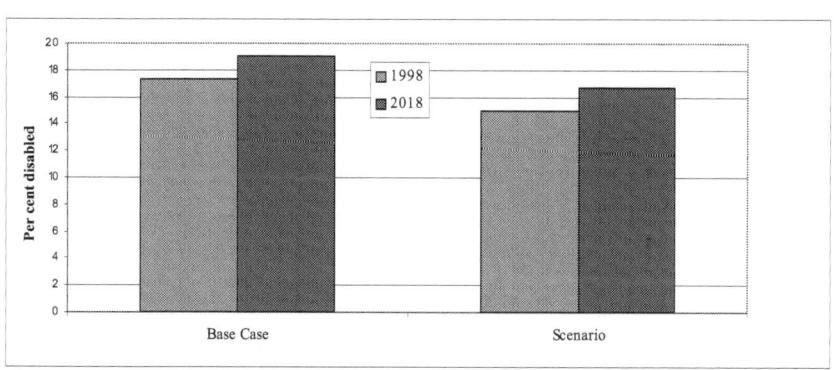

Source: simulations using DYNAMOD.

Figure 17: **Proportion disabled by health state, Base case and Scenario, 1998 and 2018**

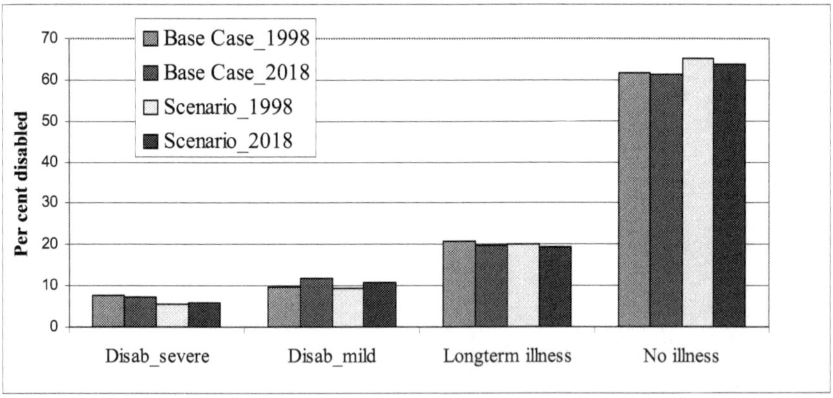

Source: simulations using DYNAMOD.

These patterns indicate a significant improvement in quality of life for those with deferred disability under the scenario, and may lead to more people being able to keep working and/or to live independently.

11.3.2 Health care costs

Total health costs in Australia were estimated at A$60.8 billion in 2000-01, with around 70 per cent of that funded by government. This was equivalent to A$3,153 per capita (AIHW, 2002 pp.5, 13).

Cost estimates in this Chapter are based on recently released disease-based expenditure data for 2000-01 (AIHW 2004). The diseases we grouped together for costing purposes include: cardiovascular disease, neoplasms, musculoskeletal conditions and 'other' (infectious & parasitic, respiratory, diabetes mellitus, endocrine, nutritional & metabolic disorders, mental disorders, digestive system, genitourinary, skin diseases, congenital anomalies).

Of particular importance to this project is that these cost data are available by age group. Age is important because most functionally impaired people are persons aged over 50 years. Also, for people over 50 the costs associated with treatment increase rapidly

(Figure18).

However, these disease-based expenditures do not cover all health costs associated with

disability. The per person disease-based average costs amount to only 78% of the per

capita health costs – that is A$2,684 compared with A$3,153. As a result, the findings

reported in Table 9 are underestimates.

Figure 18: **Expenditure on selected diseases* in 2000-01**

($/person)

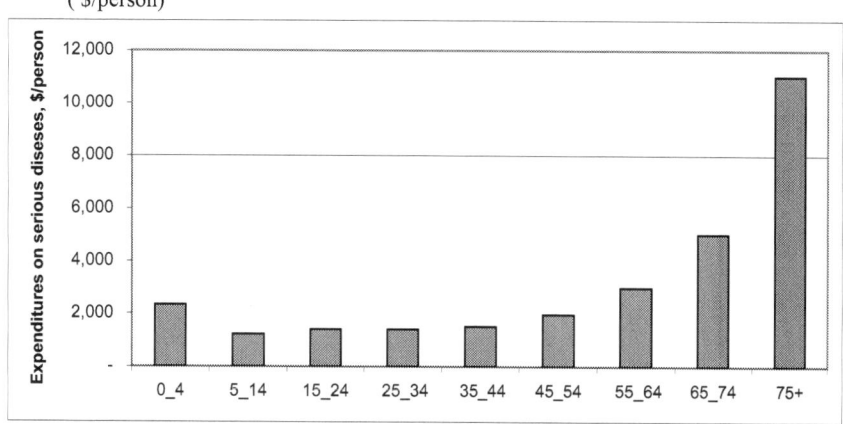

* Includes cardiovascular disease, neoplasms, musculoskeletal conditions and 'other' (infectious
& parasitic, respiratory, neonatal causes, diabetes mellitus, endocrine, nutritional & metabolic,
mental disorders, digestive system, genitourinary, skin diseases, congenital anomalies).
Source: AIHW (2004, Table 7)

Table 9 shows that deferred disability under the scenario was estimated to have saved in

1998 around a A$1 billion in health care expenditures (A$1.5 billion in 2018) – in

constant 2000-01 dollars.

In this Chapter we did not consider several of the non-monetary benefits arising from

the scenario – such as improved quality of life for those who are no longer disabled

under the scenario, and for the many unpaid carers – mainly family and friends – who

provide informal assistance to the disabled. In 2000-01 the value of unpaid welfare

services provided in households was estimated at A$29 billion (AIHW 2003b). While caring for people with a disability was only part of the overall task, the value of the

benefits of the scenario to unpaid carers would clearly be considerable.

Table 9 –Health expenditures* on the disabled by age, 1998 and 2018

Age group	Base Case $million a	Scenario $million b	Difference in expenditures $million (a-b)	Per cent change in expenditures % 100*(a-b)/a
		1998		
0_4	135	70	65	48.3
5_14	180	144	36	20.0
15_24	465	428	36	7.8
25_34	750	726	24	3.2
35_44	544	515	29	5.3
45_54	883	622	261	29.6
55_64	1,155	787	368	31.9
65_74	2,307	2,175	131	5.7
75+	5,914	5,796	118	2.0
All	12,333	11,263	1,070	8.7
		2018		
0_4	141	89	52	36.9
5_14	138	84	54	39.3
15_24	221	120	101	45.5
25_34	574	508	66	11.5
35_44	720	736	- 16	-2.2
45_54	1,385	1,095	290	21.0
55_64	1,988	1,462	526	26.5
65_74	3,611	3,394	217	6.0
75+	9,947	9,714	233	2.3
All	18,726	17,202	1,524	8.1

* Disease-based, including cardiovascular disease, neoplasms, musculoskeletal conditions and 'other' (infectious & parasitic, respiratory, neonatal causes, diabetes mellitus, endocrine, nutritional & metabolic disorders, mental disorders, digestive system, genitourinary, skin diseases, congenital anomalies).
Sources: DYNAMOD simulations, AIHW (2004) and ABS (2002b).

11.3.3 Disability Support Pension expenditures

Another government expenditure that is estimated to grow more slowly under the

scenario than under the Base case is Australia's Disability Support Pension. This pension provides income support to people with a disability who are unable to work full-time. Between 1980 and 2000, the number of Disability Support Pension recipients nearly trebled (from 229,200 to 602,300) – ABS (2002b). The reasons provided by ABS (2002b and 2001b) for these increases include more people living alone (thus can better meet the related asset and income tests); and improvements in mortality (ie people who would have died before are now kept alive disabled). Population ageing may be another reason - Cai and Gregory (2003).

Although AIHW (2001) forecasts considerable future increases in the number disabled with a severe or profound restriction – the ones most likely to qualify for the Disability Support Pension – in this thesis our cost estimates are based on the assumption that 'past trends will continue'. As a result, our findings are likely to be underestimates.

In 2000, 602,300 people aged 15 years and over received a total of A\$5.2 billion Disability Support Pension – or A\$8634 per recipient. Assuming that in 1998 a similar number, 602,300 persons (ie 18.5% of the disabled), received a disability support pension, and that that proportion applied to the differences in the numbers disabled between the Base case and the scenario (ie 430,231 persons in 1998), then the costs saved in 1998 under the scenario (through fewer Disability Support Pension recipients) would be: A\$8,634 * 430,231 * 0.185 = A\$687 million. The corresponding estimate for 2018 - assuming constant 2000 prices - would be: A\$8,634* 468,135 * 0.185 = A \$747 million.

11.4 Discussion

The complex modelling method chosen for this thesis allowed the simultaneous estimation of a range impacts associated with implementation of the 'improved public health scenario'. In summary, the findings are that, if such a scenario were implemented, close to half a million fewer Australians would be disabled, around 180,000 life years would be saved, health care costs would be around A$1 billion lower per year and the government could save close to A$700 million on the Disability Support Pension.

The estimated health improvements and potential cost savings are considerable. If subjected to traditional cost-benefit analysis,[33] these savings in health expenditures would give an indication of the order of magnitude of what the government could spend on initiating the scenario so as to more or less 'break even' over the longer term.

The following sub-sections compare the above findings with those of similar previous studies and identify areas for possible future improvement.

11.4.1 Comparisons with findings from earlier studies

Two earlier studies reported on analyses similar to those described in this Chapter: an Australian study on socioeconomic inequalities in mortality (Turrell and Mathers, 2001 and 2002) and a British study "Inequalities in life and death: what if Britain was more equal" (Mitchell et al, 2000). In the former, Australian mortality data were analysed using the SEIFA as indicator of socioeconomic status. In the latter, a SEIFA type indicator – geographic area based and named 'social class' - was computed on the basis of variables such as income, wealth and occupation.

In this Chapter we illustrated the considerably greater complexities, and broader range of questions, that use of a dynamic microsimulation model was able to address than what had been possible in these earlier studies. While in most analyses reported in the literature – including the above two - mortality alone is used as 'proxy' for health, we were able to consider both mortality and disability – with the complex linkages that exist between mortality and disability being mathematically accounted for.

---

[33] An example of a cost-benefit study in this field is the US Perry project described in section 2.7.

Consideration of disability is an important feature, because it affects people's quality of life; reduces the number of productive years they have; and impacts significantly on health-related expenditures by individuals and governments. While many of the earlier mortality-based studies had to rely on a geographic-area-based SES indexes – which were shown to underestimate the extent of health inequalities (Chapter 5) – in this study we were able to choose from several individual-based indicators.

11.4.2 Possible future improvements

The methods used in this Chapter should be seen as a first step only since considerable improvements could be made in a number of areas.

As noted earlier, availability of longitudinal data and much better coverage in surveys of Australians aged over 65 years would lead to improved estimates. This will particularly be so in future since, with more rapid improvements in life expectancies – due for example to medical advances arising from the mapping of the human genome (section 1.1.1) – the more severe stages of chronic diseases are expected to shift towards older age groups.

A useful future extension to the analyses presented in this Chapter would be the estimation of lifetime savings – as opposed to the savings in particular years. For example, we could have estimated health expenditures over the life course, in addition to presenting the cross-sectional estimates for 1998 and 2018. This would have meant identifying cohorts of interest, and summing such savings for each cohort over every year of life.

Considering health expenditures over the life course has the advantage of accounting for the longer lives that lower SES people would have under the scenario than under the Base case. Thus, while the cross-sectional savings would occur as estimated in section 11.3, in the lifetime computations account would be taken of the additional health costs associated with people living longer under the scenario. An ability to do this arises from the dynamic and individual-based structure of DYNAMOD. Lifetime computations have not been carried out for this Chapter due to the limited scope of PhD theses. However, it will be important to conduct such analyses in future, once it becomes possible to re-estimate the model using longitudinal data.

Another possible future development would be to relate disability in the model to economic and social life-cycle events – subject to suitable data becoming available.

Also, the health cost estimates in this Chapter could be significantly improved if the disease-specific data on health care expenditures could be disaggregated by severity of illness. While in Australia this would be a complex process - since administrative data on doctor, hospital and pharmaceutical expenditures cannot readily be linked to severity of illness - it is an issue worth further investigation.

Finally, research could be carried out on whether health inequalities by socioeconomic status should be studied differently amongst older Australians than amongst those of working age. Questions that have not to date been adequately answered include: 'is the childhood, or adulthood, or post retirement SES the better predictor of health amongst people aged 65 years or more'; and 'are the geographic area-based and/or income-wealth-based indicators of SES as appropriate for retired people as for those of working age'

Chapter 12   Health and the ability of older Australians to stay in the labour force

This Chapter illustrates the potential usefulness of the enhanced dynamic

microsimulation model through a study of the impact of more older Australians staying

in the labour force - subject to individuals' own health, socioeconomic status, sex, age

and family characteristics.[34] Earlier studies on the age of retirement - such as Fields

and Mitchell (1984) for the US – covered some of these elements, but did not consider

health.

The impacts of longer working lives on individuals' earnings and on the related savings

in expenditures on the age pension are also assessed. The older Australians considered

in this Chapter are those aged 65 years or over.[35]

12.1 Recent policy initiatives and future directions

Ageing populations, combined with much improved life expectancies, have led to

'longer working lives' becoming a much discussed topic in most developed countries.

Amongst the possible policy alternatives considered is the raising of the state pension

age. While some countries already have a qualifying age for the state pension that is

above 65 years – eg 67 years in Norway (Frederiksen and Stolen, 2003) – several others

are considering proposals to do so. O'Connell (2003) reports that in Germany a working

group proposed that the statutory retirement age be increased from 65 to 70 years by

2035. It also notes that in the UK where, by 2020, the pension age will be 65 years for

---

[34] The analyses detailed in section 4.3 support our choice of this topic for an application of the enhanced model.

[35] In Australia early retirement - that is people leaving the workforce before age 65 - is an issue of considerable policy concern. While this group of older Australians is excluded from the analyses presented in this Chapter, there is no reason why they could not be the subject of a similar study in future.

everyone, proposals have been made to raise it to age 67 or 70 over the next 25 to 30 years. One conclusion by O'Connell (2003, p.5) was that:

"raising the pension age may be the only way to sustain a better state pension in future, and it fits with the potential for longer working lives as we live longer".

O'Connell (2003) lists arguments generally raised in the UK against the lifting the pension age above 65, amongst which is that many people do not want to work until they are 70. The fear that due to ill health they may not be able continue working that long, and thus may end up with no income at all, is likely to be a major reason for this. O'Connell concluded that a rise in the pension age would be more acceptable if, rather than being considered in isolation, it was presented as part of an overall review of the state pension system.

As in other developed countries, in Australia the proportion of working age persons is declining and that of the retired population increasing (Treasury 2002; Treasurer 2004). In the next decade or so some 4 million 'baby boomers' are expected to join the 2 million Australians currently retired.

Earlier the Australian government initiated several policies leading to the gradual alignment of the pension age for men and women to 65 years. Regarding the situation in 1998, the available statistics suggest that there was little incentive – and possibly little opportunity - for people who reached or were above the age pension age to remain in the workforce (section 12.3.2). More recently the government asked older Australians to keep working longer (Howard, 2003) and started to introduce policies more in line with the work preferences of older persons (Treasury 2004). These include access to superannuation by those aged 65 or over who wish to remain in the labour force (but at reduced hours of work). Several recent initiatives concern 65 to 74 year olds. The extension of working lives simulated in this Chapter could arise not only from government initiatives such as the lifting of the age pension age, but also from developments such as more favourable and flexible labour market conditions and/or general improvements in health.

12.2 Aims

If a proportion of currently retired Australians could be persuaded to remain longer in the labour force, the financial benefits to individuals would be considerable and government expenditures on the retired would be reduced. However, ill health will limit the number of older people able to work longer. With over 80 per cent of Australians aged 65 years or more having at least one long term chronic illness (Walker et al, 2003), it is likely that many in that age group will be unable to continue working.

The main aims of this application are to establish how important health is in the decision to retire; what financial consequences longer working lives have for individuals and the government; and how that situation would change if the health at the population level in Australia could be improved.

The next section describes the modelling work carried out specifically for this Chapter. Details of the scenarios simulated are in section 12.4.

12.3 Modelling the employment status of 65-70 year olds

This section documents the building and the validation of the new Work_65-70 module that was added to DYNAMOD specifically to study issues related to the possible extension of older Australians working lives. We selected the 65-70 age group for closer study, because this group is most likely to be affected by proposed policy changes such as the lifting of the pension age beyond 65 years (section 12.1). The choice of 70 years as an upper limit was strengthened by the fact that beyond that age poorer health - and other effects of ageing - were expected to lead to a considerable reduction in the number of hours worked.

12.3.1 Data and methodology

To model the employment status of older Australians in a changed job and regulatory environment, we used the 1998 Disability survey unit record files (ABS 1999a). The advantages of that nationwide survey over other ABS surveys are that it is not restricted to households, has a better coverage of older age groups, and has information on ill health and its severity (Chapter 3).

Two major tasks needed to be carried out to model the employment status of older Australians in different work and health environments. To study the first one - the estimation of the likely work patterns of this older age group under the changed environment - we used logistic regression techniques. For the second - the imputation of that work pattern onto each individual in DYNAMOD - so that it reflected that individual's personal and family characteristics – we used logistic regression and the Monte Carlo method.

12.3.2 Choice of variables in explaining work patterns

For the 65-70 age group, we considered that people had extended their period of employment if they worked more than 15 hours per week. Thus, in what follows 'work' refers to working more than 15 hours per week.

Studies have shown that the major determinants of employment status are age - Cai and Kalb (2004); Green and Leeves (2003) - own health, others' health (such as spouse), sex (see Table A9.1) and SES (see ABS 1999c). When estimating the probability that 65-70 year olds will continue to 'work', we considered these factors as explanatory variables from amongst the variables available in the 1998 Disability survey, together with whether there was one or more dependent.

From amongst the SES indicators available in the 1998 Disability survey, we chose the geographic area-based SEIFA index of socioeconomic disadvantage. This was because we expected the SEIFA to be less highly correlated with employment status than the available income-based indicators of SES.[36] Also, we chose SES at age 55 – rather than current SES – because the SEIFA quintile of those retired is in general considerably lower than the SEIFA quintiles of people of the same age still working. Thus, SES at age 55 is a more appropriate indicator of socioeconomic status of the 'working' 65-70 year olds than their current SES.[37]

One difficulty presented by the patterns observed in the Disability survey was that in 1998 only a small proportion (10%) of 65-69 year olds worked 15 hours or more per week. This 10% corresponded to a sample of 160 individuals only, which proved to be too small to extract work patterns by health, SES, sex, spouse and dependent(s). As a result, to model the probability of 65-70 year olds working more than 15 hours per week, we chose a younger age group – one that still had most of its members in the workforce. Also, Appendix A9 shows that beyond age 54 most survey respondents - 59% of 55-64 year olds and 88% of 65-69 year olds - gave the 'retired' or 'too old' response as to why they were not looking for work, rather than reasons such as own or others' ill-health. Thus, the 1998 survey data for those aged 55+ could not be used to study what the work patterns of 65-70 year olds might be in future under different employment environments.

After examining work-related patterns in the Disability survey (Appendices A7 and A9), we chose the 1998 employment patterns of 45-54 year olds as an example of what might occur amongst 65-70 year olds under a changed job and regulatory environment.[38] That is we assumed that, within each 'health-SES-age-sex-spouse-dependent' cell, the work patterns of 65-70 year olds in DYNAMOD will be those

---

[36] The reason for this is that people with a job tend to have considerably higher incomes than people who are retired.

[37] SES at age 55 is indicated by the Income_Wealth measure in DYNAMOD.

[38] The Disability survey indicated that, in 1998, people started retiring from age 55 onwards – with 69% 'working' amongst 45-54 year olds, but only 49% amongst 55-59 year olds and 26% amongst 60-64 year olds.

observed in 1998 for 45-54 year olds. This assumption can be relaxed once suitable data becomes available.[39]

12.3.3 Logistic regression for the probability of working

The aim of this section is to estimate an equation for the probability of working, for use in DYNAMOD when determining which 65-70 year old will have 'working' status in each year of the model's simulation phase.

Logistic regression was applied to the 1998 Disability survey data to assess the probability p_i that an individual of given characteristics x_i would work more than 15 hours per week:

$$p_i = \text{prob(work=1} \mid x_i) = e^{\eta}/(1+ e^{\eta}) \qquad \text{(Equation 1)}$$

where

$$\eta = \mu + a*A + b_1*I_1 + b_2*I_2 + b_3*I_3 - (b_1+b_2+b_3)I_4 + c*sex + d*SP + e*Dep +$$
$$f_1*SES_1 + f_2*SES_2 + f_3*SES3 + f_4*SES_4 - (f_1 + f_2 + f_3 + f_4)*SES_5$$

with   A=1 for 45-49 year olds and A=0 for 50-54 year olds;

I_1=1 for 'No illness'; I_2=1 for 'Long term illness'; I_3=1 for 'Disability_mild restriction'; I_4=1 for 'Disability_severe restriction', with each being zero otherwise;

sex is 0 for males and 1 for females;

SP is 1 if there is a spouse and 0 otherwise; [40]

---

[39] Plans are underway to initiate such collection of more appropriate data on the work characteristics of 65+ year olds, and then possibly carry out an application similar to that of Chapter 12 as a separate policy-relevant exercise, using specially obtained funding.

[40] Although we constructed a spouse's health varaiable in the Disability survey, we were only able to consider whether the individual had a spouse or not - due to the small size of the 45-54 year old dataset (5134 records – 3902 'with spouse' and 1232 'without spouse').

Dep is 1 if there is dependent(s) and 0 otherwise;

SES (=SEIFA_Q at age 55) is a 1 to 5 categorical variable. $SES_1 = 1$ for the most disadvantaged quintile, etc.

Using Disability survey data on 45-54 year olds, the parameter estimates produced by weighted[41] logistic regression using the SAS programming language were:

μ=0.7661;   a=0.1211; b_1=1.0325; b_2=0.7476; b_3=-0.4987;   c=-1.3484;

d=0.2335;   e=-0.0199; f_1=-0.6597; f_2=-0.158; f_3=0.0413; f_4=0.2824.

The univariate results in Table 10 show that 'own health' and 'SEIFA quintile' had the greatest explanatory power (each being over 50% concordance, and 'own health' having by far the greatest Likelihood Ratio Chi-square). Sex was the next most important (with 40% per cent concordance, while 'age', 'spouse' and 'dependent' were about equally important (each with close to 30% per cent concordance). While age would normally be expected to be more important, in these analyses we only considered 45-54 year olds (that is two categorical classes: 45-49 and 50-54 year olds) and within that range the effect of age was only moderate.

As expected, for a dataset of that size (5134 individuals), the results were statistically highly significant (p<0.0001). All variables considered contributed to goodness of fit. The multivariate results in Table 10 show that the three most important variables – own health, socioeconomic status and sex – explained most of the variations observed, with the 'per cent concordant' statistic being 77.5 with these three variables, compared with 78.8 with all the variables.

Table 10: **Logistic regressions, 45-54 year olds, variables influencing whether 'working',^ 1998**

---

[41] Regressions were carried out 'weighted' because DYNAMOD – into which results from the regression equation are to be imputed - is a full population model.

Independent variables	Likelihood Ratio Chi-square (df)[#]	% concordant*
Univariate		
age - categorical	9728 (1)	28.8
sex	167751 (1)	40.0
SEIFA quintile	98078 (4)	52.3
own health	248468 (3)	52.9
spouse	24323 (1)	27.6
dependent(s)	12584 (1)	26.1
Multiple regressions (adding variables in order of importance)		
own health, SEIFA quintile	308528 (7)	68.8
own health, SEIFA quintile, sex	496915 (8)	77.5
own health, SEIFA quintile, sex, age	502640 (9)	78.2
own health, SEIFA quintile, sex, age, spouse	506614 (10)	78.5
own health, SEIFA quintile, sex, age, spouse, dependent(s)**	506650 (11)	78.8

degree of freedom in brackets * The per cent of predicted probabilities that were concordant with the responses observed in the survey ^ All results were statistically significant (p<0.0001). **This specification is Equation 1 detailed in section 12.3.3, together with the related estimated coefficients.
Source: 1998 Disability Survey

12.3.4 Imputing of 'work' status in the main model

To impute 'work' status in DYNAMOD we first used the above logistic regression equation (Equation 1) to estimate the probability p_i that a particular 65-70 year old would 'work'. Next we simulated the decision to work using a Monte Carlo approach, drawing a random number, z, from a uniform distribution over the interval [0, 1], and comparing it with the estimated probability pi .

In each year of the simulation year the person is then assigned a status of 'working' when $z <= pi$. The method of re-assigning a 'work' status to 65-70 year olds each year was chosen because of the unavailability of longitudinal data from which transition probabilities could be estimated. While in Chapter 8 we did estimate health transition probabilities from cross sectional data, in the case of employment by 65-70 year olds

suitable cross sectional data was lacking due to most people in that age group currently

being retired.

While the year-by-year method of assignment does not accurately depict what happens

to individuals over the life course, the aggregate estimates – such as the proportion of

65-70 year olds 'working' – are a reasonable reflection given the large sample sizes

embedded in DYNAMOD (8,396 persons aged 65-70 years in 1998 and 14,504 in

2018).

12.3.5 Validation

To validate the new Work_65-70 module, we carried out a random check on the

probability of 'working' predicted by Equation 1 to assess whether it had been correctly

applied to each 65-70 year old persons in DYNAMOD, when imputing their work

status. Broad-based validation comparing 1998 aggregate patterns from DYNAMOD

simulations with patterns in the 1998 Disability survey was reported in Chapter 9.

12.4 Description of the Base case and Scenario simulations

The scenario simulated is 65-70 year olds extending their working lives. One key

assumption is that the work choices of 65-70 year olds will in future follow those made

by 45-54 year olds in 1998. The reason for adopting this assumption is that, in the

available statistics, very few people 'work' after age 65. In the 1998 Disability survey

sample only 160 65-70 year olds 'worked' – representing 10% of the population

(section 12.3.2). This proved to be too small to extract work patterns by health, SES,

sex, spouse and dependent(s). This assumption is likely to result in the predicted

numbers 'working' being an over-estimate.

Another key assumption is that the 1998 health pattern of 65-70 year olds - by age, sex, SES and family type cells – remains unchanged over time. This seems a reasonable assumption, given that the positive impact of improved medical technology is likely to be offset by increases in the proportions of the overweight population.

The simulations are carried out under two different alternatives regarding population health:

- **Base case:** whereby the work pattern changes occur in an environment where health inequalities by socioeconomic status are those observed in 1998; and

- **Improved Health Scenario**: whereby the work pattern changes occur in an environment where the health of all Australians – in terms of mortality and disability rates - is lifted to that of the most advantaged 20% of the population.[42]

The results are presented in the next four sections. Section 12.5 compares the 1998 Base case 'health and work' results for 65-70 year olds with those obtained from the 1998 Disability survey for 45-54 year olds. Some of these comparisons can be seen as part of the validation of the enhanced DYNAMOD model. Sections 12.6 to 12.8 present findings for 1998 and 2018 under both the Base case and the scenario – in terms of the number of 65-70 year olds in each health state; the numbers that would be able and willing to work more than 15 hours per week; the earnings of those who remained in the workforce; and the subsequent savings on age pension expenditures by government.

12.5 Results: health and employment of 45-54 year olds versus 65-70 year olds

---

[42] For disability, this means that in the input data to DYNAMOD the 31.4% disabled in the most disadvantaged SEIFA quintile – and the 25.9%, 23.8%, 20.6% disabled in SEIFA quintiles 2, 3 and 4 respectively – will all be lowered to 17.8% (ie to match the proportion disabled in the most advantaged SEIFA quintile).

To assess whether the model results were in line with expectations, the health and employment patterns in the 1998 Disability survey were compared with those in DYNAMOD under the Base case. Figure 19 shows the distribution by health state of the population aged 45-54 years in the survey and that of the 1998 DYNAMOD population aged 65-70 years.

Figure 19 shows that, while over 80% of the 45-54 year old survey population had no disabilities – and thus no related impact on their ability to 'work' - that proportion was considerably lower for the DYNAMOD 65-70 year olds (around 70%). As a result, in 1998, the proportion working amongst 45-54 year olds was higher than that amongst 60-70 year olds (Figure 20).

Figure 19: **Distribution of the 45-54 and 65-70 populations by health state, ABS Survey and DYNAMOD, Base case, 1998**

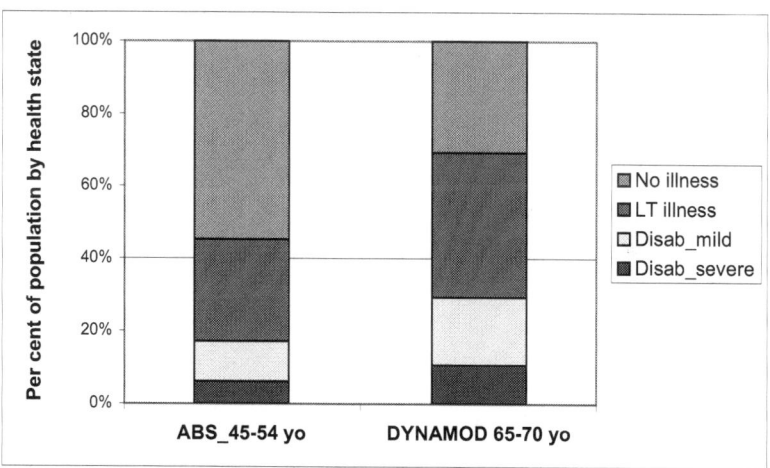

Sources: ABS 1998 Disability Survey (1999a) and DYNAMOD simulations

Figure 20: **Per cent of 45-54 and 65-70 populations 'working' by health state,* ABS survey and DYNAMOD, Base case, 1998**

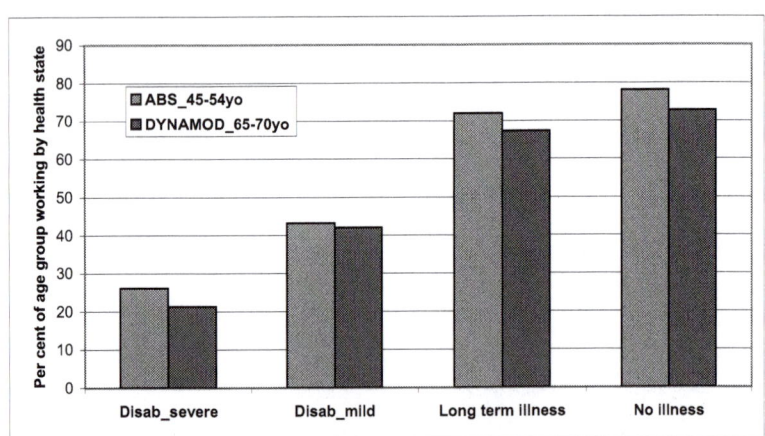

* Based on a logistic regression equation for 'work' by health state only.
Sources: ABS 1998 Disability Survey (1999a) and DYNAMOD simulations

Because we used Equation 1 with a single explanatory variable (ie health state) when constructing Figure 20, these findings on 'work' can be interpreted as arising uniquely from the poorer health of 65-70 year olds than that of 45-54 year olds. A key finding from Figure 20 is that, due to poorer health in older ages, 7% less of the DYNAMOD population of 65-70 year olds were 'working' than of the population of 45-54 year olds.

This finding has consequences for superannuation and age pension policies, in that account needs to be taken of the smaller and smaller proportion of the population healthy enough to be able to 'work' as people age. Another conclusion is that 'prevention' of the more severe stages of chronic illnesses has the potential to significantly increase the proportion 'working' in a given older age group – hence the inclusion in this Chapter of the Improved Health Scenario.

12.6 Results: predicted population of 65-70 year olds and the proportion working

Table 11 shows the estimated population of 65-70 year olds by health status under the Base case and the Improved Health Scenario in 1998 and 2018. It indicates that for 1998 the model generated a total of 864,800 persons aged 65-70 years. The corresponding population published by the ABS is 817,000 persons – indicating a reasonable alignment between the DYNAMOD results and publicly available benchmark data.

Table 11 also shows that - as expected - the total number of 65-70 year olds are similar under the Base case and the scenario.[43] The improvements in population health manifest themselves by there being *less* disabled under the scenario than under the Base case (29.6% less for severe disability in 1998 and 16.6% in 2018), and *more* with neither illness or disability (17.5% in 1998 and 28.3% in 2018).

The smaller difference in 2018 arises mainly from the upward drift in the proportion disabled built into the model (section 9.2).

Table 12 shows how many 65-70 year olds are predicted to 'work' under both the Base case and the scenario. In 1998, 516,200 persons aged 65-70 years are estimated to work more than 15 hours per week under the Base case. This compares with 55,000 persons aged 65-69 years working the same hours per week in the 1998 Disability survey (ABS 1999a). After subtracting these 55,000, the implementation of 'extending working lives' policies and related societal changes was estimated to result in 450,000 more 65-70 year olds remaining in the workforce in 1998 (around 800,000 in 2018) than in the absence of such changes.

---

[43] The small difference between these estimates arises from the probabilistic nature of DYNAMOD and the number of deaths being lower under the Improved Health Scenario than under the Base case.

Table 11: **Persons* aged 65-70 years by health status, Base case and Scenario, 1998 and 2018**

	65-70 year olds		
	Base case	**Scenario**	**Difference**
	(a)	(b)	(b-a)/a
	'000	'000	%
1998			
Disabled	252.9	178.0	-29.6
severe restr'n	91.5	63.3	-30.7
mild restr'n	161.4	114.6	-29.0
Long term illness	345.7	373.9	8.2
No illness or disability	266.3	312.9	17.5
All health states	864.8	864.8	0.0
2018			
Disabled	419.5	350.0	-16.6
severe restr'n	145.5	95.1	-34.7
mild restr'n	274.0	254.9	-7.0
Long term illness	655.0	622.0	-5.0
No illness or disability	419.4	538.2	28.3
All health states	1493.9	1510.2	1.1

* NOTE: numbers in Table may not add up due to rounding. Also, the total number of persons under the Base case and the scenario are slightly different in 2018 due mainly to less people dying under the scenario.
Source: DYNAMOD simulations

Table 12 also shows that there would be around 7% more 65-70 year olds 'working' under the scenario than under the Base case. This is mainly due to there being less disabled working under the scenario than under the Base case – 29% less in 1998 and 16% less in 2018. As before, the smaller 16% difference in 2018 arises mainly from the upward drift in the per cent disabled built into the model (section 9.2).

Table 12: **Number of 65-70 year olds working more than 15 hours per week, Base case and Scenario, 1998 and 2018**

	65-70 year olds		
	Base case	**Scenario**	**Difference**
	(a)	(b)	(b-a)/a
	'000	'000	%
1998			
Disabled	87.2	62.4	-28.5
severe restr'n	19.5	17.3	-11.1
mild restr'n	67.8	45.1	-33.4
Long term illness	234.6	259.7	10.7
No illness or disability	194.4	230.9	18.8
All health states	516.2	553.0	7.1
2018			
Disabled	155.2	130.5	-15.9
severe restr'n	37.0	26.5	-28.4
mild restr'n	118.2	104.0	-12.0
Long term illness	454.3	452.8	-0.3
No illness or disability	313.1	401.2	28.1
All health states	922.7	984.5	6.7

* NOTE: numbers in Table may not add up due to rounding.
Source: DYNAMOD simulations.

12.7 Results: earnings of 65-70 Year Olds

The earnings of 65-70 year olds were based on what 45-54 year olds who worked more than 15 hours per week earned, and for whom wage or salary was the main source of income (ABS 1999a). We used the person level 'total weekly cash income' variable in the survey (Table 13). The earnings of 60-64 year olds would have been more appropriate, there were too few respondents in the survey in that age group who had wages or salaries as their main source of income. For most, their income came mainly from government (age pension). However, it is possible to compare the earnings in

Table 13 with the median weekly cash incomes of respondents aged 65 years or over who provided information on their incomes from 'wages, salaries, own business or a partnership' (ABS 1999c, Table 26). Incomes from these sources amounted to $340 per week for the disabled and $420 per week for the people without disability. While these earnings are considerably lower that those in Table 13, they include incomes earned working less than 15 hours per week, and income earned without being in the labour force – eg from own business or a partnership.

Table 13 shows that in 1998 the mean weekly cash income of 45-54 year olds was $737 from wages or salaries. Assuming that this age group drew this salary 52 weeks in the year, then the corresponding income is $38,000 a year – an income well above the average earnings of all age groups working more than 15 hours per week ($32,500). This is as expected, because people's incomes tend to increase as their career progresses with age, and because those with skills/education who command higher salaries are more likely to have a job.

Table 13: **Mean weekly cash incomes of 45-54 year olds who worked more than 15 hours per week and whose main source of income was from wages and salaries, by health state** (1998 dollars)

Age	45-49	50-54	45-54
1998	$	$	$
Disabled, severe restr'n	640	603	625
Disabled, mild restr'n	659	664	662
Long term illness	742	746	744
No illness or disability	742	746	744
All health states	737	738	737

Source: 1998 Disability survey, unit record files – ABS (1999a).

Table 13 also shows that in both the 45-49 and 50-54 age groups the earned incomes of the disabled - while well above the age pension[44] - were significantly lower than the earned incomes of the non-disabled.

Using the DYNAMOD generated estimates of the numbers of 65-70 year olds who worked more than 15 hours per week (Table 12) and the mean earnings data in Table 13, the annual earnings of the working 65-70 year olds under the Base case and the scenario are presented in Table 14. These estimates were prepared assuming that the same weekly earnings were received 52 times in the year.

Table 14 indicates that under the Base case the earnings of persons aged 65-70 years would have been $19.8 billion in 1998 ($35.4 billion in 2018) – in 1998 constant prices.

Table 14: **Annual earnings* of 65 to 70 year olds, Base case and Scenario, 1998 and 2018** (1998 dollars)

	65-70 year olds		
	Base case (a)	**Scenario** (b)	**Per cent change** (b-a)/a
	$ million	$ million	%
1998			
Disabled			
severe restr'n	633	562	-11.1
mild restr'n	2333	1553	-33.4
Long term illness	9078	10046	10.7
No illness or disability	7519	8934	18.8
All health states	19784	21193	7.1
2018			
Disabled			
severe restr'n	1202	860	-28.4
mild restr'n	4070	3581	-12.0
Long term illness	17577	17517	-0.3
No illness or disability	12114	15521	28.1
All health states	35361	37729	6.7

* Assumes that the weekly earnings reported in the 1998 Disability survey (ABS 1999a) occurred 52 times in the year.   ** Defined as whether working more than 15 hours per week.
Sources: DYNAMOD simulations for the numbers working more than 15 hours per week (Table 12); Table 13 for the person level estimates of earnings.

---

[44] As at September 1998, the single age pension was $178.65 per week. For couples it was $149.05 each per week – Department of Family and Community Services (2004).

Accounting for the 55,000 persons who would have worked without the Base case changes, the 1998 estimate becomes $17.7 billion. Under the scenario, the earnings of 65-70 year olds would be around 7% higher than under the Base case ($1.4 billion higher in 1998 and $2.4 billion in 2018).

12.8 Results: expenditures on the age pension for 65-70 year olds

We initially assumed that, for every person working under the Base case and the scenario, the government would save on the age pension. This is because currently only a very small proportion of 65-70 year olds work more than 15 hours per week, and because their earnings are likely to be well above the age pension (section 12.7).

To be able to estimate the impact of longer working lives on government expenditures on the age pension, we first examined the related statistics published by the Department of Family and Community Services (1999, p.5). For 1999 these indicate that:

- out of the 1.7 million Australians aged 60 years or more who received the age pension, close to 0.5 million were aged 65-69 years (27.9%);

- the proportion of singles amongst all Australians receiving the age pension was 47.3% and of couples 52.7%; and

- 68.2% received the maximum pension rate and 31.8% a reduced rate.

The first point shows that people in the age group we are studying – 65-70 years olds – accounted in the late 1990s for close to a third of all age pensioners. Also, comparing the 1.7 million receiving the age pension with ABS population statistics, around 70% of Australians aged 60 years or more received the age pension in 1999.

The average full and part pension rates were obtained from Treasury (1999, Table 6).

Based on the total age pension expenditure in 1997-98 ($13,141 million), we found that,

on average, the part pension rate amounted to around half of the full pension rate.

In view of the above statistics, we made some assumptions when estimating the savings

on the age pension under the Base case and the scenario (Table 15).

Table 15: **Assumptions made when estimating age pension expenditures on 65-70 year olds, Base case and Scenario, 1998 and 2018**

Proportion of the 65-70 year old population with the age pension	70.0%
Proportion of age pension customers - 'single' rate	47.3%
Proportion of age pension customers - 'couple' rate	52.7%
Proportion of age pension customers - full pension	68.2%
Proportion of age pension customers - part pension	31.8%
Ratio of part pension to full pension	0.5

Sources: Department of Family and Community Services (1999) and Treasury (1999)

We also assumed that the average earnings of 65-70 year olds who 'worked' under the

Base case and the scenario were equal to those shown in Table 13 – and were thus not

eligible for the age pension (section 12.7).

Based on these assumptions, Table 16 shows that the total saving on the age pension in

1998 was estimated at $2.6 billion under the Base case (4.6 billion in 2018) – in

constant 1998 prices. When adjusted for the 55,000 persons[45] who would have 'worked'

without any changes in the current situation, this $2.6 billion reduces to $2.2 billion -

equivalent to 17% of the government's 1997-98 expenditure on the age pension.

Table 16 also shows that under the Improved Health Scenario, the government would

save about $4.9 billion (1998 dollars) on the age pension in 2018 – an amount that is

around 7% greater than under the Base case.

---

[45] The number of 65-69 year olds in the Disability survey (ABS 1999a) who worked more than 15 hours per week in 1998 was around 55,000.

Table 16: **Potential savings on the age pension of 65 to 70 year olds if their employment patterns* were similar to that of 45 to 54 year olds in 1998, 1998 and 2018** (1998 dollars)

	65-70 year olds		
	Base case	**Scenario**	**Difference**
	(a)	(b)	(b-a)/a
	$ million	$ million	%
1998			
Disabled	435	312	-28.5
severe restr'n	97	86	-11.1
mild restr'n	338	225	-33.4
Long term illness	1171	1296	10.7
No illness or disability	970	1153	18.8
All health states	2577	2760	7.1
2018			
Disabled	775	651	-15.9
severe restr'n	185	132	-28.4
mild restr'n	590	519	-12.0
Long term illness	2268	2260	-0.3
No illness or disability	1563	2002	28.1
All health states	4605	4914	6.7

* Defined as working more than 15 hours per week.
Sources: DYNAMOD simulations for the numbers working; Department of Family and Community Services (2004 and 1999) for age pension statistics.

12.9 Results: comparing the Base case and Scenario results

Potential savings on the age pension under the scenario were estimated to be around 7% greater than under the Base case. For example, the additional earnings of 65-70 year olds were around $19.8 billion in 1998 and $35.4 billion in 2018, compared with $21.2 and $37.7 billion under the scenario - Table 14. The related savings on the age pension under the Base case were $2.6 billion in 1998 ($4.6 billion in 2018), compared with $2.8 billion ($4.9 billion) under the scenario - Table 16.

This implies that considerably greater financial benefits would arise from effective government incentives for 65-70 year olds to remain in the workforce - combined with improved job availability for that age group – than from improved population health (arising from the lifting of the health of all Australians to that of the most advantaged 20% of the population). However, improved public health will have many benefits not accounted for in this Chapter. As seen in Chapter 11, under the same assumptions as for the scenario in this Chapter, close to one million fewer Australians would be disabled, over 180,000 life years would be saved, health care costs would be of the order of A$3 billion lower and the government could save about A$1 billion on the disability support pension. Thus, the scenario simulated in this Chapter should be only seen as accounting for that scenario's impact on the likely work patterns of 65-70 year olds.

12.10 Discussion

The study method chosen for the thesis allowed us to model the decision to retire as a function of each individual's own health, socioeconomic status, age, sex and family composition. An additional 450,000 persons aged 65-70 years were estimated to remain in the workforce - with the related earnings totalling up to $20 billion in 1998 ($35 billion in 2018) and savings by government on the age pension of around $2 billion ($4 billion in 2018). The study method chosen also allowed the estimation of the combined impacts of the 'longer working lives' scenario (Chapter 11) and the 'narrower health inequalities scenario' (Chapter 12).

This application demonstrated the importance of including health into discussions about the desirability of older Australians extending their working lives. It used a novel analytical method that allowed the *simultaneous* consideration of the many variables –

such as health, life expectancy, earning capacity, socioeconomic status and family composition - that impact on the decision to remain in the workforce after age 65. The study also provided estimates of the financial consequences of longer working lives for individuals and government.

However, our analyses have several limitations. Probably the most important ones are the lack of historical statistics on the employment patterns of 65-70 year olds - due to most Australians in this age group being at present retired; the lack of data on how older Australians are likely to respond to recent and likely future government initiatives which encourage the extension of working lives; and the uncertainly about job availability for those 65-70 year olds who are willing and able to continue working under the changed regulatory environment. A further limitation is that the increase in GDP resulting from 65-70 years working – which is expected to be small - was not taken into account.

Other limitations arise from the assumptions and exclusions that are inevitably made in studies of this kind. One such assumption is that in future the reluctance by Australian employers to retain or hire older workers[46] would disappear. While some improvements in the acceptance of older workers are already apparent, it is unlikely that such reluctance would disappear completely – suggesting that our findings could be an over-estimate.

Another assumption that may result in an over-estimate is that the 65-70 year olds working more than 15 hours per week would work at that intensity for 52 weeks in a year. In this respect our findings can easily be adjusted for people working only part of the year.

---

[46] ABS (2003b, p.16) found that, amongst the unemployed, 30% of 45-54 year olds said that being 'considered too old by employers' was their main difficulty in finding work, with this proportion nearly doubling for the 55+ age group (59%).

For example, if 65-70 year olds were assumed to 'work' for only 26 weeks in a year, then the earnings and age pension cost estimates would need to be halved. The tendency to over-estimation due to these two assumptions is offset by the exclusion in our analyses of older Australians who worked less than 15 hours per week; of people retiring between ages 55 and 65;[47] and, for the 2018 results, the much slower upward drift modelled in disability rates than what past trends indicate.

Another exclusion is the non-consideration of unpaid carers – mainly family and friends – who in 2000-01 provided informal assistance to the disabled valued at A$29 billion (AIHW 2003b). The more older people remain in the workforce, the more this informal assistance will diminish, putting greater pressure on governments to replace the informal unpaid care with formal paid services for the disabled and the frail old.

---

[47] Treasurer (2002) contains a scenario with higher full time labour force participation of 45-64 year old men. "Overall, higher full-time labour force participation of older men, under this scenario, would reduce projected government spending by 0.25 per cent of GDP by 2041-42, principally by increasing GDP. This reduced spending is mainly in health and Age Pensions. However, this only captures first order effects, and does not capture any potential second order effects, such as changes in health or health service use of the additional older workers who remained in the workforce for longer." – p.63.

PART 3: OVERALL CONCLUSIONS

Chapter 13   Conclusions and possible future developments

Section 1.1.1 noted that, in the post 'mapping of the human genome' era, the capacity to study the complex links between disease and mortality patterns over the life course, and to analyse the financial and equity effects of possible responses, were particularly important. The following sections summarise the extent to which these issues had been achieved in this thesis, and the improvements that could be made in future.

13.1 Conclusions

13.1.1 PART 1: Modelling the links between health and socioeconomic status

The thesis has demonstrated that the health-SES link can be successfully built into a dynamic microsimulation model. Its model building aims, as set out in section 1.1.2, had been achieved, with several novel methodologies having been developed in the process. These are detailed below.

Model building achievements

The basis of the model building tasks carried out for this thesis is an existing dynamic microsimulation model for Australia, DYNAMOD. The state-of-the-art techniques adopted at the time of its development are still chosen for new models currently being developed internationally (section 2.6). The Australian model is based on good quality – though mainly cross-sectional – data (section 1.4). It has been validated against published official statistics (section 9.1); and there is extensive publicly available documentation on various aspects of its model building phase (footnote 4, section 1.4).

Dynamic microsimulation models have the considerable advantage of bringing data together in a coherent fashion from many unrelated sources, so that individuals' life courses can be studied in a more comprehensive fashion than with traditional methods (section 1.2.1).

Two new modules were incorporated into DYNAMOD: one adding a socioeconomic dimension to the health aspects of the original model (Health_SES module) and the other taking account of the progressively deteriorating health status of Australians as they age (Health State Transitions module).

There were a number of *challenges* associated with the building of these two new modules. The *first* concerned the gaining of an in-depth understanding of the structure of the model; the variables, parameters and functions it contained; and the numerous interconnection that existed between them (section 1.5.3). This challenge was overcome by studying the model's extensive documentation; by gaining familiarity with the model's code (initially requiring the learning of the C programming language); and eventually by gaining sufficient depth of understanding of the code to allow its modification when attaching the new modules.

The *second* challenge was to find suitable data for building the new modules. One dataset chosen for the Health_SES module was the AIHW extract for mortality – by age and sex; SEIFA as the indicator of SES; and causes of deaths (the latter allowing separate identification of mortality rates for the able-bodied and the disabled). The dataset chosen for the disability variable was the 1998 Disability survey (ABS, 1999a) – by age, sex, and three possible types of SES measures (the geographic-area level SEIFA, and two individual income-based indicators especially constructed for this thesis). Both data sources were sufficiently large to allow disaggregation by the variables of interest to this project (full population for the AIHW data and 40,000 records for the ABS data). Both were of high quality (section 3.4). The 1998 Disability survey was also used in the building of the Health State Transition module.

However, these data sources were not ideal for all our needs. In particular, the Disability survey only provided cross sectional data, when longitudinal data would have been preferable, especially for the Health State Transition module. A novel methodology developed to overcome the lack of longitudinal data is described in Chapter 8.

The *third* challenge was to build and validate the new modules, that is: prepare the input data required associated with these in a format acceptable to DYNAMOD (Chapter 6); impute socioeconomic status and disability by age, sex and SES to DYNAMOD's Base data(section 7.1); re-work the DYNAMOD C code to allow incorporation of the new modules (section 7.2, Chapter 8 and TableA1.1 in Appendix A1); and validate each of the new modules by aligning them to external benchmark statistics (Chapter 9).

Novel approaches

Because in this thesis health was modelled within a considerably broader context than in other dynamic microsimulation models (section 2.6), and because of the scarcity of longitudinal data in Australia, creative approaches had to be developed. These include:

- moving away from the traditional mortality-based indicator of health, towards a methodology able to account for disability over the life course, together with its eventual impact on mortality (Chapter 4)

  - allowing a re-focussing of analyses toward 'what quality of life people have while they are alive' rather than 'how long people live for';

- accounting for the health-mortality relationship by socioeconomic status, as well as by the traditional age-sex variables generally considered in the literature (Chapter 6);

- identifying inadequacies in the official data available in Australia, such as the finding that household-based health surveys - which exclude the institutionalised – distort actual health patterns, especially for people aged 70 years or more. As a result, only the disability survey - which does include the institutionalised - was used in this thesis (section 3.3);

- showing that the health-SES patterns traditionally reported in the mortality-based literature no longer hold with income/wealth based indicators of SES, and when population ageing is accounted for (Chapter 5); and that

  - individual-level income-based SES indicators are more appropriate for studies of income inequalities than the a geographic area-based SEIFA. This is because age, which was found to be the single most important factor affecting disability, is not accounted for in the SEIFA (section 5.7.1);

- developing more complex indicators of socioeconomic status than those generally used in the literature. In particular, in this thesis we took account of wealth as well as the traditional family income and family size variables (Chapter 7);

- taking account of the progression of chronic diseases over the life course when developing the SES indicator of health/disability status (Chapter 8). This allowed:

  - the study of the way health status interacted with 'functionality', which in turn could be linked to people's ability to remain in the labour force (Chapter 12);

  - the study of the financial consequences for individuals and for government of a narrowing of health inequalities (Chapter 11); and

- the developing of a novel methodology for overcoming the lack of Australian longitudinal data when estimating transition probabilities from one health state to the next (section 8.3).

13.1.2 PART 2: Applications of the enhanced model

The additional aim of the thesis – that is the application of the enhanced model to topical issues - has also been achieved. Two novel and policy relevant – though at this stage illustrative – applications of the enhanced dynamic microsimulation model were described in Chapters 11 and 12. The broad ranging questions addressed in these applications illustrate the considerable benefits that arose from choosing to graft the new modules onto a comprehensive existing model, rather than build two stand-alone models to address the topics of Chapters 11 and 12.

The application in Chapter 11 simulates the impact of a narrowing in health inequalities in Australia as health is lifted nationally to the level currently enjoyed by the most affluent 20% of the population. The findings were that, if such a policy change were implemented, close to half a million fewer Australians would be disabled, around 180,000 life years would be saved, health care costs would be around A$1 billion lower per year and the government could save close to A$700 million on the Disability Support Pension.

These findings show that, through use of the modelling approach chosen for this thesis we were able to provide results for health benefits and for cost savings simultaneously. They also show that the estimated cost savings arising from implementation of the policy change are considerable. If subjected to traditional cost-benefit analysis,[48] these cost savings could indicate the order of magnitude of what the government could spend

---

[48] An example of a cost-benefit study in this field is the US Perry project described in section 2.7.

on initiating the policy change simulated, so as to more or less 'break even' over the longer term.

The application in Chapter 12 quantifies the likelihood and the financial impacts of Australians aged 65-70 years continuing to work in future, under a number of assumptions. In this application, the study method chosen for the thesis allowed us to model the decision to retire as a function of each individual's own health, socioeconomic status, age, sex and family composition. An additional 450,000 persons aged 65-70 years were estimated to remain in the workforce - with the related earnings totalling up to $20 billion in 1998 ($35 billion in 2018) and savings by government on the age pension of around $2 billion ($4 billion in 2018).

The study method adopted for the thesis also allowed the estimation of the combined impacts of the 'longer working lives' scenario (Chapter 11) and the 'narrower health inequalities scenario' (Chapter 12).

This application has consequences for superannuation and age pension policies, since it quantifies the smaller and smaller proportions of the population healthy enough to be able to 'work' as people age. It also shows the beneficial consequences of the 'prevention' of the more severe stages of chronic illnesses by estimating the increase in the number of older Australians healthy enough to remain in the labour force.

13.2 Possible future developments

Chapter 10 discusses several limitations of the research presented in this thesis. Some of these concern limitations generally associated with modelling, since a model can never be more than a simplified version of the real world. Some other limitations, however, could in future be overcome, and had only been listed as a limitation within the context of a PhD thesis – for example, the researching of the most appropriate alignment and validation methodologies (sections 10.1 and 10.4) and sensitivity testing (section 10.3). These tasks could be considered to be possible future developments.

On the methodology side, the techniques used to align dynamic microsimulation models are still being researched (section 10.1). There is considerable scope to identify in future methodologies and their applications that informed modellers as to which technique could be accepted as 'best practice' in which particular application.

Areas for possible future development were also mentioned in several other Chapters. One example is the extension of the scenario analyses to estimation of health impacts and expenditures over the life course (section 11.4.2). This is an area where, in future, better use of the 'lifetime' capabilities of dynamic microsimulation (section 1.4) could be harnessed in Australia.

In addition, future studies could make use of several variables available in existing data sources, but not used in this thesis due to the limited scope of the project. These include 1998 Disability survey variables, such as the 'main disabling conditions; the related 'duration of the main disabling condition'; and information on comorbidities (Appendix A7, section A7.5). If necessary, additional disease-related information could be imputed from the ABS's 'causes of death' statistics, or from its National Health Surveys (Appendix A2, sections A2.1 and A2.4.1). Such developments would allow the disaggregation of the disability-related results presented in Chapters 11 and 12 down to impacts at the disease level.

With more longitudinal and other data expected to become available in Australia, considerable further improvements could arise from re-assessing the way DYNAMOD is structured and the programming language its code is written in (sections 1.4 and 1.5.3). One example concerns the need – due to current data difficulties - to use SEIFA-based SES indicator for the disability-mortality equations, and a family income-based one for the health transition probabilities (section 5.8). Linking of Census data over time and statistically matching Census and mortality data – as currently planned by the ABS – may overcome this problem in future, with patterns of income over the life course becoming available. Also, a relatively simple improvement to the enhanced model would be to add a module estimating the probability that a person with a certain health state would be institutionalised (eg to enter a nursing home). Such an improvement would allow an assessment of whether that person could continue to live independently. Using DYNAMOD's ability to track family relationships, such an extension would also open up the possibility of studying a range of aged care issues– eg the extent to which care could be given informally by a spouse or children (Walker 1997). While carrying out such an improvement, the recent trend toward de-institutionalisation – with rapid increases in the use of shared accommodation arrangements – could also be taken into account.[49]

Another possible area for future research is the development of a methodology for modelling the cumulative impact of various factors affecting health over the life course – one such factor being low SES and its duration early and in later life. This is a particularly complex but important area, and the actual carrying out of such research would be subject to data availability.

Another extension to the model could be the harnessing of the suitability of dynamic microsimulation models to track intergenerational patterns – an area of particular policy concern amongst lower SES groups (section 2.2).

Improvements could also be made in future to the applications of the enhanced model. For example, the health cost estimates in section 11.4.2 could be significantly improved if the disease-specific data on health care expenditures could be disaggregated by

---

[49] Over the period 1981 to 1998, the proportion of the disabled in cared accommodation declined considerably, despite the numbers disabled increasing from 453,000 in 1981 to 955,000 in 1998 (Madden and Anderson, 2004).

disease severity. While in Australia this would be a complex process - since administrative data on doctor, hospital and pharmaceutical expenditures cannot readily be linked to individuals' functionality - it is an issue worth further investigation. Another improvement would be the subjecting of many of the the key assumptions adopted in this thesis to sensitivity testing.

Finally, the model could be further improved if the relationship between the health of older Australians and their socioeconomic status was better understood. Questions that have not been adequately answered to date include: 'is the childhood, or adulthood, or post retirement SES the better predictor of health amongst people aged 65 years or more'; and 'are the geographic area-based and/or income-wealth-based indicators of SES as appropriate for retired people as for those of working age'.

160

References

Abello, A., King, A. and Robinson, M., 2002, *Demographic Projections with DYNAMOD-2*, National Centre for Social and Economic Modelling, Technical Paper no. 21, University of Canberra.

ABS (Australian Bureau of Statistics), 2003a, *National Health Survey: Australia 2001, User Guide*, Cat No 4363.0, Canberra.

—— 2003b, *Household Income and Income Distribution*, Cat No 6523.0, 2003, Canberra.

—— 2002a, *Disability, Ageing and Carers (Survey of)*, www.abs.gov.au/Ausstats@nsf/lookupMF/NT00020EDA, accessed 24 September.

—— 2002b, *Australian Social Trends 2002 - Income and Expenditure – Income Support: Trends in Disability Support* – AusStats, downloaded 4/04/03.

—— 2001a, *Government Benefits, Taxes and Household Income: 1998-99*, Cat No 6537.0, Canberra.

—— 2001b, *Accounting For Change In Disability And Severe Restriction*, 1981–1998, Working Papers in Social and Labour Statistics, No 2001/1.

—— 2000a, 1998 *Disability Ageing and Carers: Disability and Long Term Health Conditions*, Cat no. 4433.0, Canberra.

—— 2000b, *1998-99 Household Expenditure Survey: User Guide*, Cat no. 6527.0, Canberra.

—— 2000c, *Australian National Accounts: Concepts, Sources and Methods*, Cat no. 5216.0, Canberra.

—— 1999a, *Disability Ageing and Carers, 1998*, Confidentialised Unit Record Files.

—— 1999b, *Disability Ageing and Carers, 1998, User Guide*, Cat no. 4431.0, Canberra

—— 1999c, *Disability Ageing and Carers1998: Summary of Findings*, Cat no. 4430.0, Canberra

—— 1999d, *Deaths of Older persons*, Special article, Cat no 3101.0, Canberra

—— 1998a, and earlier issues *Causes of Deaths, Australia*, Cat no. 3303.0, Canberra

—— 1998b and earlier issues, *Deaths, Australia*, Cat no. 3302.0, Canberra

—— 1998c, *1996 Census of Population and Housing: Socioeconomic Indexes for Areas*, Information Paper Cat no 2039.0, Canberra

—— 1996a, *1995 National Health Survey: Users' Guide*, Cat no. 4363.0, Canberra

—— 1996b, *1995 National Health Survey: Summary of Results*, Cat no. 4364.0, Canberra

161

—— 1996c, *Projections of the Populations of Australia, States and Territories: 1995–2051*, Cat no. 3222.0, Canberra.

—— 1995, *1993-94 Household Expenditure Survey: User Guide*, Cat no. 6527.0, Canberra.

—— 1993a, *Causes of Death, Australia, 1992*, Cat no 3303.0, Canberra.

—— 1993b, *Disability Ageing and Carers1993, Summary of Findings*, Cat no 4430.0, Canberra.

—— 1993c, *Disability Ageing and Carers1993*, Confidentialised Unit record Files.

—— 1991a, *1989-90 National Health Survey: Users' Guide*, Cat no. 4363.0 and associated questionnaire

—— 1991b, *Socioeconomic Indexes for Areas*, Information Paper, Cat. no. 2912.0, Canberra.

—— 1990, *1983 National Health Survey Questionnaire A2* (unpublished ABS document).

—— 1982, *Australian Health Survey 1977-78*, Cat No 4323.0 (which includes the related questionnaires)

Acheson, D. 1998, *Independent Inquiry Into Inequalities in Health Report*, London, The Stationary Office, 1998.

Ackerman, D. 2000, 'Do the Maths: High School Mathematics Classes and the Lifetime Earnings of Men', presented at *Australian National University, Seminar for Economists* series, 16 November.

AIHW (Australian Institute of Health and Welfare), 2005, *Australian Health Inequalities 2: Trends in Male Mortality by Broad Occupational Group*, AIHW Bulletin No. 25

——2004, *Health System Expenditure on Disease and Injury in Australia 2000-01*, Health and Welfare Expenditure Series No. 19, Canberra.

—— 2003a, *Disability Prevalence and Trends*, Canberra.

—— 2003b, *Australia's Welfare 2003*, Canberra.

—— 2002, *Health Expenditure, Australia 2000-01*, Canberra.

—— 2001, *Australia's Welfare 2001*, Canberra.

Andrews, G and Clark, M (2000), *Predictors of crucial social and health outcomes in the Australian Longitudinal Study of Aging (ALSA)*, paper presented at Panel Data and Policy Conference, May 1-3, Canberra.

Antcliff, S, 1993, *An Introduction to DYNAMOD:a Dynamic Microsimulation Model*, National Centre for Social and Economic Modelling, , DYNAMOD Technical Paper no. 1, University of Canberra.

Antcliff, S., Bracher, M., Gruskin, A., Hardin, A. and Kapuscinski, C, 1996, *Development of DYNAMOD: 1993 and 1994*, National Centre for Social and

Economic Modelling, Dynamic Modelling Working Paper no 1, University of Canberra.

Arber, S. 1996, 'Integrating Nonemployment Into Research on Health Inequalities', *Int J Health Serv*, 26: 445-481.

Armitage and Berry, 1994, *Statistical Methods in Medical Research*, Blackwell Science, Oxford (UK).

Attanasio, O. and Emmerson, C. 2003, 'Mortality, Health Status and Wealth', *Journal of the European Economic Association*, Vol. 1, 4:821-850, June.

Bækgaard, H., 2002a, *Micro-Macro Linkage and the Alignment of Transition Processes*, National Centre for Social and Economic Modelling, Technical Paper No. 25, University of Canberra.

—— 2002b, *Modelling the Dynamics of the Distribution of Earned Income*, , National Centre for Social and Economic Modelling, Technical Paper no. 24, University of Canberra.

Bartley, M. and Owen, C. 1996, 'Relation Between Socioeconomic Status, Employment and Health During Economic Change, 1973-93', *British Medical Journal*, 313:445-449, 24 August.

Bartley, M, Power, C, Blane, D, Davey Smith, G and Shipley, M 1994, 'Birth Weight and Later Socioeconomic Disadvantage: Evidence from the 1958 British Cohort Study', *British Medical Journal*, 309:1478 (3 December)

British Medical Journal 1997, 'Poverty and equity matter', no. 314, 22 February, editorial, first page.

Bosma, H., Marmot, M., Hemingway, H., Nicholson, A., Brunner, E. and Stansfeld, S. 1997, 'Low Job Control and Risk of Coronary Heart Disease in Whitehgall II (Prospective Cohort) Study', *British Medical Journal*, 22 February, 314:558.

Bradbury, B.,Norris, K. and Abello, D. 2001, *Socioeconomic Disadvantage and the Prevalence of Disability*, Social Policy Research Centre, SPRC Report 1/01 prepared for the Victorian Department of Human Services, University of New South Wales, Sydney.

Brown, L., Walker, A., Waters, A. and Thurecht, L. 2002, *Funding of High Cost Biotechnology and Other Innovative Targeted Therapies under the Pharmaceutical Benefits Scheme*, National Centre for Social and Economic Modelling, Position Paper, 27 February.

Brown, L. Jackson, Steven B. Caldwell, and Stephen. A. Eklund, 1995, 'How Fee and Insurance Changes Could Affect Dentistry: Results from a Microsimulation Model', *Journal of the American Dental Association*, Vol. 126, April, pp. 449-459

—— 1992, 'Microsimulation of Dental Conditions and Dental Service Utilization', pp. 111-116 in Anderson, J.G. (ed.) *Proceedings of Simulation in Health Care and Social Services Conference,* Society for Computer Simulation, San Diego.

Brunner, E. 1997, 'Socio-economic Determinant of Health: Stress and the Biology of Inequality', *British Medical Journal,* Vol.314, pp. 1472-1476.

Butler, J.R. 1996, 'A microsimulation model of the Australian health sector: design issues', Paper presented at the *Australian Conference of Health Economists,* Coffs Harbour, July.

Cai, L. and Kalb, G. 2004, *Health Status and Labour Force Participation: Evidence from the HILDA Data,* Working Paper No 04/2004, Melbourne Institute of Applied Economic and Social Research, University of Melbourne.

Cai, L. and Gregory, R., 2003, 'Inflows, Outflows and the growth of the Disability Support pension (DSP) Program, *Australian Social Policy 2002-03, pp 121-143,* Canberra.

Caldwell, S. and Morrison, R. 2000, 'Validation of longitudinal dynamic microsimulation models: experience with CORSIM and DYNACAN'. In: Mitton, L., Sutherland, H., and Weeks M (eds) *Microsimulation Modelling for Policy Analysis,* Cambridge, UK.

Caldwell S. 1996 'Health, Wealth, Pensions and Life Paths: The CORSIM Dynamic Microsimulation Model'. In A. Harding (ed.) *Microsimulation and Public Policy.* Amsterdam: North Holland.

Caldwell, S et al., 1993, *The NIDR/CORSIM Model: Final Report To NIDR* (in Six Volumes).

Clarke, P. and Smith, L. 2000, 'More or Less Equal? Comparing Australian Income-Related Inequality in Self-Reported Health with Other Industrialised Countries', *Australian and New Zealand Journal of Public Health,* Vol 24, No 4, pp 370-3

Crimmins, E. M. 1996, 'Mixed Trends in Population Health Amongst Older Adults', *J Gerontol* 51B: S23-S25.

Department of Family and Community Services 2004, *Rates of Pension,* accessed from www.facs.gov.au/guide/ssguide/52210.htm on 14 March 2004

—— 1999, *Income Support Customers: a Statistical Overview,* Canberra.

Department of Housing and Regional Development 1995, *Household and Family Forecasting Models — A Review,* AGPS, Canberra.

Davey Smith, G. 2002, *Health Inequalities: lifecourse approaches,* Policy Press, University of Bristol, UK.

Davis, B., Heathcote, C, O'Niell, T. and Puza, B. 2002, *The Health Expectancies of Older Australians,* Research School of Social Sciences, Australian National University, Working Papers in Demography No 87.

Doherty, P., 2001, 'The Map of Life', *Kenneth Myer Lecture* delivered at the National Library of Australia, Canberra, December. See www.abc.net.au/rn/talks/bbing/stories

Draper, G., Turrell, G. and Oldenburg, B. 2004, *Health Inequalities in Australia: Mortality*. Health Inequalities Monitoring Series No. 1. Australian Institute of Health and Welfare Cat. No. PHE 55, Canberra.

Dunn, C., Sadkowsky, K. and Jelfs, P. 2002, *Trends in Deaths: Analysis of Australian data 1987-1998 with updates to 2000*, Mortality Surveillance Series No 3, Cat No PHE 40, Australian Institute of Health and Welfare, Canberra.

Dunnell, K., 1995, 'Population Review: (2) Are We Healthier?', *Population Trends*, Vol 82, Winter 1995, pp. 12-18, published by the UK Government Statistical Service

Eckermann, S. 1992, Projected health expenditure and ageing: revised methodologies, Paper presented at the PHA Conference, Canberra, September.

Evandrou, M., Falkingham, J., Johnson, P., and Rake, R., 2001, *Simulating Social Policy for an Ageing Society: A Research Agenda*, Discussion Paper 1. ESRC-Sage Research Group, London.

Fields, G and Mitchell, O. 1984, The Effects of Social Security Reforms on Retirement Ages and Retirement Incomes, *Journal of Public Economics*, 25: 143-59.

Forum on Research Study Design, 1999, *Forum on Research Study Design — Report*, National Centre for Epidemiology and Population Health, Australian National University, Canberra, 5 May.

Fredriksen, D and Stolen, M. 2003, "Possible Ways to Moderate the Future Pension Burden in Norway", *7th Nordic Conference on Microsimulation Models*, 12-13 June, Helsinki, Finland.

Glasson, W. 2004, (President, Australian Medical Association), *Speech to the National Press Club*, 14 July 2004, Canberra.

Glover, J., Harris, K. and Tennant, S. 1999, *A Social Health Atlas of Australia*, 2nd edition, Volume 1, Public Information Unit, University of Adelaide, South Australia.

Giele, J. and Elder, G. (eds). 1998, *Methods of life course research: Qualitative and quantitative approaches*. London: Sage.

Glover, J., Rosman, D. and Tennant, S. 2004, 'Unpacking Analyses Relying on Area-based Data: are the assumptions supportable?', *International Journal of Health Geographics,* 3:30, 9 December.

Gordon, D., Shaw, M., Dorling, D. and Davey Smith, G. (eds) 1999, *Inequalities in Health: The Evidence*, Independent Inquiry into Inequalities in Health chaired by Sir Donald Acheson, The Policy Press, Bristol, UK.

Graetz, B. 1993, 'Health Consequences of Employment and Unemployment: Longitudinal Evidence for Young Men and Women,' *Soc Sci Med,* 36: 715-724.

Gregg, P. and Machin, S. 2000, 'The Relationship Between Childhood Experiences, Subsequent Educational Attainment and Adult Labour Market Performance', paper presented at the *Panel Data and Policy Conference* convened by the Department of Family and Community Services, 1-3 May, Canberra.

Gregory, R. and Hunter, B. 1995, *The Macro Economy and the Growth of Ghettos and Urban Poverty in Australia,* Centre for Economic Policy Research, Discussion Paper No 325, Australian National University, April.

Green C. and Leeves, G. 2003, 'The Incidence and Consequence of Worker Displacement in Australia', *Australian Economic Papers*, Vol 42, Issue 3, p. 316, September.

Goss, J., Eckermann, S., Pinyopusarerk, M. and Wen, X. 1994, Economic perspective on the health impact of the ageing of the Australian population in the 21st Century, Paper presented at the Conference of the Australian Population Association, Australian National University, Canberra, September.

Harding, A. and Greenwell H, 2001, 'Trends in Income and Expenditure Inequality in the 1980s and 1990s' -- Paper Presented to the *30th Conference of Economists*, Perth, Australia, 24 September.

Harding, A, Percival, R., Schofield, D. and Walker, A. 2002, '*The Lifetime Distributional Impact of Government Health Outlays'*, *Australian Economic Review*, vol. 35, no. 4.

Harding, A, King, A. and Kelly, S. 2002, *Trends in the Incomes and Assets of Older Australians,* Discussion Paper 58, National Centre for Social and Economic Modelling, University of Canberra.

Harding, A. (ed.) 1996, *Microsimulation and Public Policy*, North Holland, Amsterdam.

Harris, E., Webster, I. and Lee, P. 1998, 'Unemployment and Health: the Healthcare System's Role', *Medical Journal of Australia*, 168, 16 March.

Hayen, A.,Lincoln, D., Moore, H. and Thomas, M. 2002, 'Trends in Potentially Avoidable Mortality in NSW', *NSW Public Health Bulletin*, Vol 13 No 11-12; 226-36

Hayes, L. 2002, Letter to the Editor: Socioeconomic Inequalities in All Cause and Specific Cause Mortality in Australia: 1985-1987 and 1995-1997, *Int J Epidemiol* 2002;31:257-258.

Headey, B. and Wooden, M. 2004, *The Effects of Wealth and Income on Subjective Well-Being and Ill-Being*, Working Paper No 03/2004, Melbourne Institute of Applied Economic and Social Research, University of Melbourne.

Health Canada, Microsimulation Modelling and Data Analysis Division, *2000-2001 Annual Report*, Ottawa.

Healy, E., 2000, 'The Shift to Long Working Hours: a Social and Political Crisis in the Making', *People and Place*, vol. 8, No 1, pp38-50

Hemingway, H. and Marmot, M. 1999, 'Psychsocial Factors in the Aetiology and Prognosis of Coronary Heart Disease: Systematic Review of Prospective Cohort Studies', *British Medical Journal*, 29 May, 318:1460-1467.

Hemingway, H., Stafford, M., Stansfeld, S., Shipley, M. and Marmot, M. 1997, 'Is the SF-36 a valid Measure of Change in Population Health? Results From the Whitehall II Study', *British Medical Journal*, 15 November, 315:1273-1279.

HM Treasury, 1999, *Persistent Poverty an Lifetime Inequality: the Evidence*, Occasional paper no. 10, Centre for Analysis of Social Exclusion, UK.

Hancock, R., Comas-Herrera, R., Wittenburg, R. and Pickard, R. 2002, 'Who will pay for long term care in the UK? Projections linking macro and microsimulation models." Paper prepared for International Network of Research on Elder Care, Hannover, 8-9 February.

Horton, I. 1998, *Beginning Visual C++ 6*, Wrox Press Ltd, Birmingham, UK.

Howard, J.,Prime Minister, 2003, *Address to Symposium on Mature Age Employment*, Sydney, 27 August.

Hyndman, J., Holman C., Hockey R., Donovan R., Corti B., Rivera J. 1995, 'Misclassification of Social Disadvantage Based on Geographic areas: comparison of postcode and collector's district analyses', *Int J Epidemiol*, **24:**165-176.

Jargowsky, P. 2003, *The ecological fallacy*, Political Economy Working Paper 04/03, School of Social Sciences, University of Texas, Dallas.

Johnson, T., 2001, *Nonlinear Alignment by Sorting*, Strategic Forecasting unpublished paper, New York.

Kelley, A. and Pohl, I. 1990, *A Book on C: Programming in C*, Benjamin/Cummings Publishing Company, Redwood City, California.

Kelly, S., Farbotco, C. and Harding, A. 2004, *Income, Superannuation and Debt Pre and Post Retirement*, AMP-NATSEM Income and Wealth Report, March.

Kelly, S. 2003, *Estimating the Wealth of Australians: a New Approach Using Microsimulation*, PhD thesis, University of Canberra, unpublished.

Kelly, S. 2002, 'Simulating Future Trends in Wealth Inequality', Paper presented at the 2002 Australian Conference of Economists, 3 October, Adelaide.

Kernigan, B. and Ritchie, D. 1988, *The C Programming Language*, Prentice Hall, New Jersey.

King, A., Walker, A. and Harding, A, 2001, 'Perspectives on Australian Retirement Incomes', *Australian Economic Review* Vol 34, No 2, pp 155-69.

King, A., Walker, A. and Bækgaard, H. 2002, *Modelling Overseas Migration in DYNAMOD-2*, National Centre for Social and Economic Modelling, Technical Paper no. 22, University of Canberra.

King, A., Bækgaard, H., and Robinson, M, 1999a, *The Base Data for Dynamod-2,* National Centre for Social and Economic Modelling, Technical Paper No. 20, University of Canberra.

—— 1999b, *Dynamod-2: An Overview*, National Centre for Social and Economic Modelling, Technical Paper No. 19, University of Canberra.

Kirkwood, T., 2001, 'The End of Age: New Directions', *Reith Lectures* (lecture 5-transcript), British Broadcasting Commission, UK. See www.bbc.co.uk/radio4/reith2001

King's Fund, 1999, *Local Inequalities Targets*, King's Fund Publications, UK.

Klevmarken, N. 1997, 'Behavioural Modelling in Micro Simulation Models: a Survey', Working Paper 1997:31, Department of Economics, *Uppsala University*.

Kuh, D. and Ben-Shlomo (eds) , 1997, *A Life Course Approach to Chronic Disease Epidemiology*, Oxford University Press, Oxford, UK.

Lee E., 1974, A computer program for linear logistic regression analysis, *Computer Programs in Biomedicine*, 80 -92.

Lynch, J, Kaplan, G and Shema, S 1997, 'Cumulative impact of sustained economic hardship on physical, cognitive, psychological and social functioning', *New England Journal of Medicine*, vol. 337, no. 26, p. 188.

Lynch, J., Davey Smith, G. Harper, S., Hillemeier, M., Ross, N., Kaplan, G. and Wolfson. M. 2004, 'Is Income Inequality a Determinant of Population Health? A Systematic Review', *The Milbank Quarterly*, Vol. 82, No. 1, pp. 5–99

McCain, M and Mustard, F. 2002, *The Early Years Study Three Years Later*, The Founders' Network of the Canadian Institute for Advanced Research, Toronto, Canada.

—— 1999, *Early Years Study*, Government of Ontario, Canada.

McCracken K., 2001, 'Into a SEIFA SES cul-de-sac?' *Aust NZ J Public Health*, 2001; 25: 305-6.

McCullagh, P. and Nelder J. 1989, *Generalized linear models*, Second Edition, London, Chapman and Hall.

McDowell, I., Newell, C. 1996, *Measuring Health: a Guide to Rating Scales and Questionnaires*, Oxford University Press.

Madden, R. and Anderson, P. 2004, 'A Decade of Disability Data',. Australian Institute of Health and Welfare Seminar, 13 July 2004, Canberra.

Manton, K and XiLiang G, (2001), 'Changes in the prevalence of chronic disability in the United States black and nonblack population above age 65 from 1982 to 1999'. *Proceedings of the National Academy of Sciences*, Vol 98, No11, pp6354-59.

Marmot, M. 1998, 'Contribution of psychosocial factors to socio-economic differences in health', *Millibank Quarterly*, vol. 76, no. 3, pp. 403–48.

Marmot, M, Smith, G., Stanfeld, S. et al 1991, "Health Inequalities Among British Civil Servants: The Whitehall II Study', *Lancet*, 337 (8754): 1387-1393.

Marmot, M, and McDowall M., 1986, Mortality Decline and Widening Social Inequalities. *Lancet*; ii:274-76.

Mathers, C., Vos, T. and Stevenson, C, 1999, *The Burden of Disease and Injury in Australia*, Australian Institute of Health and Welfare.

Mathers, C., 1995, *Health Differentials Among Australian Children*, Australian Institute of Health and Welfare, Health Monitoring Series No 3, Canberra.

Mathers, C. and Schofield, D. 1998, 'The Health Consequences of Unemployment: the Evidence', *Medical Journal of Australia,* 168: 178-182.

Mejer, L and Siermann, C, 2000, "Income Poverty in the Europan Union: Children, Gender and Poverty Gaps", *Statistics in Focus*, Eurostat.

Mitchell, R., Shaw, M. and Dorling, D., 2000*, Inequalities in Life and Death: What if Britain Were More Equal?*, published for the Joseph Rowntree Foundation by the Policy Press, Bristol, UK.

Morell, S.,Taylor, R. and Kerr, C. 1998, 'Unemployment and Young People's Health', Medical Journal of Australia, 168, 16 March.

Morell, S.,Taylor, R., Quine, S. et al, 1994, 'A Cohort Study of Unemployment as a Cause of Psychological Disturbance in Australian Youth', *Soc Sci Med*, 38:1553-1564.

Morrison, R. 2001, 'Make It So!', unpublished research note.

—— 1999, 'The Proof of the Policy Model Is In ...', paper presented at the *Public Policy Analysis and Management: Global and Comparative Perspectives Conference,. 4 –6 November, Washington, D.C.*

National Research Council 1991, *Improving Information for Social Policy Decisions: The Uses of Microsimulation Modelling*, National Academy Press, Washington, DC.

Nelissen, J., 1996, *Medical Consumption, Contributions to and Redistribution by the Dutch Health care System: An Analysis by Means of Microsimulation*, Worc Report 96.10.004/2.

Neufeld, C. 2000, 'Alignment and Variance Reduction in DYNACAN', in Gupta, A and Kapur, V.(eds) *Microsimulation in Government Policy and Forecasting*, North-Holland, Elsevier.

Newman, J. 1999, Minister for Family and Community Services, *The Future of Welfare in the 21st Century*, 29 September, Canberra.

Neill, A. 1977, *Life Contingencies*, Heinemann Professional Publishing, Oxford.

Newman, J, Minister for Family and Community Services 1999a, *The Future of Welfare in the 21st Century*, Media release, Canberra, 29 September.

NSW Health Department, 1997, *The Health of the People of New South Wales*, Report of the Chief Health Officer, , December, Sydney.

O'Connell, A., 2003, *Raising the State Pension Age: an Update*, Pensions Policy Institute Discussion Paper, UK.

O'Donoghue, C. and Sutherland, H. 1999, Accounting for the family in European income tax systems, *Cambridge Journal of Economics*, 23: 565-598.

O'Donoghue, C. 2003, *Alignment Methods*, unpublished communication, UK.

—— 2001 (ed), 'Special Issue on Dynamic Microsimulation', *Brazilian Electronic Journal of Economics*, Vol. 4, Number Two, Recife, December 15th.

OECD (Organisation for Economic Co-operation and Development) 1998, *Health Outcomes in OECD Countries: a Framework of Health Indicators for Outcome-oriented Policy Making*, Labour Market and Social Policy Occasional Paper No 36, Paris.

—— 1996, *Policy Implications of Ageing Populations: Introduction and Overview*, OECD Working Paper no. 33, Paris.

Orcutt, G.1957, 'A new type of socio-economic system', *Review of Economics and Statistics*, Vol 58, No 2.

Orcutt, G., Greenberger, M., Korbel, J., Rivlin, A. 1961, *Microanalysis of Socioeconomic Systems: A Simulation Study*, Harper and Row, New York.

Orcutt, G., Merz, J. and Quinke, H. 1986, *Microanalytic Simulation Models to Support Social and Financial Policy*, North Holland, New York.

Oxman, T., Brekman, L., Kasl, S., Freeman, D., and Barrett, J. 1992, 'Social Support and Depressive Symptoms in the Elderly', *American Journal of Epidemiology*, Vol 135, No 4, pp 356-368.

Pamuk E, Macuk D, Heck K, Reuben C, Lochner K., 1998, *Socioeconomic Status and Health Chartbook: Health United States 1998.*, National Center for Health Statistics, Hyatsville MD.

Petterssen, T. and Petterssen, T. 2003, Lifetime Redistribution Through Taxes, Transfers and Noncash Benefits, *7th Nordic Conference on Microsimulation Models*, 12-13 June, Helsinki, Finland.

Pudney, S., Sutherland, H., 1993, *Statistical Reliability and Microsimulation: the Role of Sampling, Simulation and Estimation Errors*, Microsimulation Policy Modelling Unit paper No MU 9402, University of Cambridge, UK.

—— published as Pudney, S., Sutherland, H., 1994, 'How reliable are microsimulation estimates? An investigation of the role of sampling error in a UK tax-benefit model', *Journal of Public Economics.*

Richardson, J 1998, 'The Health Care Financing Debate' in Mooney, G. and Scotton, R.B. (eds), *Economics and Australian Health Policy*, pp. 192-213.

Richardson, J. and Robertson, I. 1999, 'Ageing and the Cost of Health Services', Proceedings of Conference on *The Policy Implications of the Ageing of Australia's Population*, Productivity Commission and Melbourne Institute, Melbourne, 18-19 March.

Ringen, S. and de Jong, P. (eds), 1999, *Fighting Poverty: Caring for Children, Parents, the Elderly and Health*, Foundation of International Studies in Social Security, Birmingham, UK .

Robine, J-M. 2001, 'Future Prospects for Human Longevity and Health', *Conference on Modelling Policy in an Ageing Europe*, London School of Economics, 11 January, UK.

Robinson, M. and Bækgaard, H., 2002, *Modelling Students in DYNAMOD-2*, National Centre for Social and Economic Modelling, Technical Paper no. 23, University of Canberra.

Robinson, W. 1950, Ecological Correlations and the Behavior of Individuals. *American Sociological Review*, Vol. 15: 351-357.

Saunders, P. 1996, Poverty, *Income Distribution and Health: An Australian Study*, Social Policy Research Centre, University of New South Wales.

—— 1990, Employment Growth and Poverty: and Analysis of Australian Experience 1983-1990, Social Policy Research Centre Discussion Paper No 25, University of New South Wales.

Schofield, D., 1996, *The Impact of Employment and Hours of Work on Health Status and Health Service Use*, Discussion Paper 11, National Centre for Social and Economic Modelling, University of Canberra.

Smith, G. D., 1997 'Socioeconomic Differentials' in Kuh, D. and Ben-Shlomo, Y. (eds) *A Life Course Approach to Chronic Disease Epidemiology*, Oxford University Press, pp.242-273.

Spielaue, M. 2002, 'Dynamic Microsimulation of Health Care Demand, Health Care Finance and the Economic Impact of Health Behaviour, Part I: Background and Comparison with Cell-based models' Report IR-02_032, *International Institute for Applied Systems Analysis*, Austria.

Stroustrup, B. 1992, *The C++ Programming Language*, Addison-Weslwy Publishing Company, 2nd edition, Reading, Massachusetts, USA

Tallis, R., 1994, 'Health Care in Old Age: an Agenda for Discussion', pp 75-88, in Marinker, M. (ed), *Controversies in Health Care Policies: Challenges to Practice*, BMJ Publishing Group.

Taylor, R. and Salkeld, G. 1996, 'Health Care Expenditure and Life Expectancy in Australia: How Well Do We Do?' *Australian and New Zealand Journal of Public Health*, Vol. 20, pp. 233-40.

Tomison, A. and Wise, S., 1999, *Community-Based Approaches in Preventing Child Maltreatment,* NCPCH Issues Paper no. 11, Australian Institute of Family Studies, Melbourne.

Treasurer, 2004, Australia's Demographic Challenges (available from www.treasurer.gov.au)
—— 2002, *'Intergenerational Report'*, Budget Paper No 5, 2002-03 Budget (available from www.budget.gov.au).

Treasury, 2004, *A More Flexible And Adaptable Retirement Income System*, Canberra.

—— 2002, *Intergenerational Report*, Budget Paper No 5, 2002-03 Budget (available from www.budget.gov.au), Canberra.

—— 1999, *1998-99 Budget Paper No 4*, accessed on www.budget.gov.au , 15 March 2004, Canberra.

Turrell, G and Mathers, C., 2000, Socioeconomic Status and Health in Australia, *MJA, Vol,* 2000: 172: 434-437.

Turrell, G and Mathers, C. 2001, Socioeconomic Inequalities in All Cause and Specific Cause Mortality in Australia: 1985-1987 and 1995-1997. *Int J Epidemiol* 2001; 30: 231-239.

—— 2002, Author response to Hayes, Letter to the Editor, *Int J Epidemiol,* 2002, 31: 257-258.

Turrell, G., Oldenburg, B., McGuffog, I. and Dent, R. 1999, *Socioeconomic Determinants of Health: Towards a National Research Program and a Policy and Intervention Agenda*, Queensland University of Technology, School of Public Health, Ausinfo, Canberra.

Vaillant, G. 2002, *Ageing Well*, Little, Brown and Company, New York.

Van Imhoff, E., and Post, W. 1998. 'Microsimulation methods for population projection.' *New Methodological Approaches in the Social Sciences, Population: An English Selection* Special Issue: 97-138.

Vinson, T. 1999, *Unequal in Life: the Distribution of Social Disadvantage in Victoria and New South Wales*, Ignatius Centre, Jesuit Social Services, August.

Wachter, K., Knodel, J.and van Landingham, M. 2001, Parental Berevement: Heterogeneous Impacts of AIDS in Thailand, Report No 01-493, Population Studies Centre, Institute for Social Research, University of Michigan.

Walker, A. and Abello, 2000, A., *Changes in the Health Status of Low Income Groups in Australia, 1977-78 to 1995*, Discussion Paper 52, National Centre for Social and Economic Modelling, University of Canberra.

Walker, A, Percival, P. and Harding, A. 2000, *The Impact of Demographic and Other Changes on Expenditure on Pharmaceutical Benefits in 2020 in Australia*, in Sutherland, H. (ed) *Microsimulation in the New Millenium: Challenges and Innovations*, Cambridge University Press. See also Discussion Paper 31, National Centre for Social and Economic Modelling, University of Canberra.

Walker, A., Kelly, S., Harding, A and Abello, A. 2003, *Does Your Wealth Depend on Good Health?*, AMP-NATSEM Income and Wealth Report, National Centre for Social and Economic Modelling, University of Canberra, March.

Walker, A. and Becker, N. 2005, 'Health Inequalities Across Socioeconomic Groups: Comparing Geographic-Area-Based and Individual-Based Indicators', *Public Health* (in press).

Walker, A. 2005 'Health Status and the Ability of Older Australians to Stay in the Labour Force, in Gupta, A, Harding, A. and Lloyd, R. (eds), *Microsimulation Modelling of Health and Aged Care*, North Holland, Elsevier (forthcoming).

—— 2004a, 'Economic and Health Impacts of Narrower Health Inequalities, Australia', refereed *Proceedings of the 3rd International Conference on Health Economics, Management and Policy*, Athens, 3-5 June 2004 (in press).

—— 2004b, 'Impact of Health on the Ability of Older Australians to Stay in the Workforce - with Possible Contributions to Economic Sustainability', *Refereed Proceedings of the Conference: 'A Future that Works - Economics, Employment and the Environment'*, University of Newcastle, 8-10 December.

—— 2003, 'Narrowing of Health Inequalities in Australia: Impacts Simulated Using a Dynamic Microsimulation Model', *7th Nordic Conference on Microsimulation Models*, 12-13 June, Helsinki.

—— 2002, 'Modeling Health Inequalities Using Dynamic Microsimulation: Statistical Issues and Future Scope' in Gulati, C., Lin Y., Mishra S. and Rayner, J. (eds), *Advances in Statistics, Combinatorics and Related Areas*, World Scientific, Singapore, pp 332-348.

—— 2001a, 'Health Inequalities and Income Distribution, Australia: 1977 to 1995', paper delivered at plenary session of the *Health Outcomes Conference*, 27-28 June, Canberra, Australia.

—— 2001b, 'Modelling Health Inequalities Using Dynamic Microsimulation: Statistical Issues', paper delivered at the 'Role of Statistics in Health' session of the *International Conference on Statistics, Combinatorics and Related Areas*, University of Wollongong, Australia, 19-21 December.

——2001c, 'Assessing Health Inequalities Using a Dynamic Microsimulation Model', paper presented at the *Health Services & Policy Research Conference*, Victoria University, Wellington, New Zealand, 2-4 December.

—— 2000a, 'Modelling Immigrants to Australia to Enter a Dynamic Microsimulation Model', in Gupta, A and Kapur, V.(eds) *Microsimulation in Government Policy and Forecasting*, North-Holland, Elsevier.

—— 2000b, '*Measuring the Health Gap Between Low Income and Other Australians, 1977 to 1995: Methodological Issues*', Discussion Paper 50, National Centre for Social and Economic Modelling, University of Canberra.

—— 1998, *Australia's Ageing Population:What Are The Key Issues And The Available Methods Of Analysis?*, National Centre for Social and Economic Modelling, Discussion Paper no. 27, University of Canberra.

—— 1997, *Australia's Ageing Population: How Important Are Family Structures?*, National Centre for Social and Economic Modelling, Discussion Paper no. 19, University of Canberra.

Wilkinson, R., 1996, *Unhealthy Societies: the Afflictions of Inequality*, Routledge, London.

Wolf, D. 2002, 'Dynamic Microsimulation of Elders' Health and Well-being,' Center for Policy Research, Maxwell School, Syracuse University, Syracuse (US), www-cpr.maxwell.syr.edu/microsim

—— 2001, 'The role of microsimulation in longitudinal data analysis',Paper No 6, Microsimulation Series, Center for Policy Research, Maxwell School, Syracuse University, Syracuse (US).

World Health Organization, 2000, *The World Health Report 2000 – Health Systems: Improving Performance*, Geneva.

World Health Organisation – Europe, 1998, *Social Determinants of Health: the Solid Facts*, Copenhagen, Centre for Urban Health.

Zaidi, A and Rake, K 2001, *Dynamic Microsimulation Models: a Review and Some Lessons for SAGE*, Discussion paper No 2, Discussion Paper, London, ESRC-Sage Research Group, London.

APPENDICES

A1 Description of DYNAMOD - original version and the Wealth module

A1.1 Original version

The material presented here is referred to in sections 1.4, and 1.5, and in Chapter 4.

The dynamic micro-simulation model to which the health module was added – DYNAMOD - was developed at the National Centre for Social and Economic Modelling, University of Canberra. Work on the model commenced in 1993. The first two versions of the model ran on a UNIX system, because at that time sufficiently powerful PCs were not as yet available. Technical documentation of the first version covered progress in the model's development during 1993 and 1994 - see Antcliff (1993) and Antcliff et al (1996).

The second phase, DYNAMOD–2, concerned the 1995 to 1999 period. Various elements of that version of the model are described in King, Baekgaard and Robinson (1999a and 1999b), Abello, Pederson and King (2000), Bækgaard (2000), Robinson and Bækgaard (2000) and King, Walker and Bækgaard (2001). The current version, DYNAMOD-3.4, runs on a PC and includes model development from 2000 onwards.

DYNAMOD is a full population model able to project the entire Australian population forward. The model's Base year dataset is based on a 1 per cent representative sample of the Australian population (150,000 persons), extracted by the Australian Bureau of Statistics from its 1986 Census. [50] The model simulates future events occurring in these persons' lives, such as births, deaths, immigration, emigration, couple formation,

---

[50] With the complete 1 per cent sample the weight for each DYNAMOD person - when estimating total population results - would be 100. However, because some records were deleted in the model's Base dataset due to Census 'non-response' – the weight attached to each person in the model is 103.

education, disability, employment, earned income, taxes, government transfers and the accumulation of wealth.

The Base data for the model involved considerable transformations of some of the Census data, and imputation of variables not provided in the Census. These latter include disability (imputed by age, sex and whether working, unemployed or not in the labour force); levels of the education variable; some elements of fertility; hours worked by full time students; and weekly earnings for all those employed. King et al (1999a) describe in detail the transformations of Census data and imputations that were carried out when developing DYNAMOD's Base data.

The model uses two methods to simulate events happening in a person's life. The first concerns *transition probabilities*, used extensively for example when simulating changes in people's labour force status. The second involves the use of *survival functions* used when modelling most demographic occurrences.

At various points throughout the simulation, the profile and other characteristics of persons are written to a history file. This allows the circumstances of an individual to be analysed either at a particular point in time (cross sectional view), or over the person's life course (longitudinal view).

The structure of the original DYNAMOD code written in the C programming language is detailed in Table A1.1 and the new programs developed for purposes of this thesis are described in section 1.5. The parts of the original DYNAMOD code that had to be modified to accommodate these new programs have been **bolded** in Table A1.1. Key DYNAMOD variables are listed in Table A1.2.

Table A1.1: **Program structure – original version of DYNAMOD**

Program identifier	Purpose	Description
	Program files	
1 Ath1prob	Tracks changes in family composition when children leave home	Computes probability of leaving home for persons in school.
2 Ath2prob		Computes probability of leaving home for persons in post secondary education
3 **Babies**	Used when new baby is born	Creates new baby. Records date of birth, sex and family links. **Allocates to baby the family's SES. Allocates initial disability status, 'disability date to' and computes initial date of death, by SES.** Initialises other DYNAMOD variables.
4 **Deathdis**	Embodies complex mathematical formulae linking disability and death	**Reads in disability_mortality data, by SES. Simulates disability_death linkages (equations in section 4.4), also by SES.** Accounts for higher life expectancies in later years of the simulation period
5 **Disab**	Processes the disability and recovery events in the crystal ball	**Adjusted to consider disability and recovery by SES**
6 **Init**	Initialises the input dataset	**Adjusted to consider disability, recovery and mortality by SES**
7 **Immig**	Processes immigrants as they enter Australia	Reads in the charactersistics of immigrants as they are added to the initial DYNAMOD population. **Adjusted to attach a socioeconomic status to immigrants, so that their disability, recovery and mortality can be simulated as a function of SES**
8 **Hf_ctrl**	Manages the buffer used to store the information in the 'history files'	**The 'History files'**, which are a record of the model's massive output, **were extended to allow consideration of variables by SES.** The 'History files' can then be analysed, using the SAS programming language, either in a cross sectional or in a longitudinal format.

9	**Death**	Processes death as specified in crystal ball	Process is carried out once time of death is reached in simulator (death recorded, Ref person, fam income etc changed). **Adjusted to allow consideration of death by SES**
10	Birth_cal	Re-arranges original birth hazard function	Makes model calibration less cumbersome. Aligns average hazard with ABS number of births by age group by year
11	Cpldiss	Processes couple dissolution	Forms two new family units of couple when dissolving the relationship
12	Cplform	Processes couple formation	Lists eligible males; matches these to potentially suitable females; records the new family unit;
13	**Crystal**	Processes the crystal ball	Records new events (eg marriage, birth), up-dates existing events (eg disability), etc. **Adjusted to allow consideration of the relevant variables by SES**
14	Demog	Processes the demographic events	Calculates the survival dates for the demographic events (eg marriage, cohabitation, pregnancy) and updates the crystal ball with the new date for the event
15	Earn_cal	Earnings calibr'n	Rearranges earnings into groups, determines which group the individual belongs to and calibrates earnings
16	Edprob	Probabilities re education	Sets up a series of logit equations that compute the probabiliy of a person transiting : year 10 - 11, 11 – 12, 12-uni, 'not study'-'post 2y' (function of age, sex, ethnicity)
17	Educ	Simulates the education of individuals	Generates the educational transitions from year 10 - 11, 11 – 12, 12-uni, 'not study'-'post 2y', using logit equations (see above); calibrates these transitions; accounts for students working – incl. their earnings
18	Educ_align	Processes alignment of education	Controls alignment mechanism for the simulation of education against historical data; updates history files
19	Educ_femcs	For females, processes exiting or continuing course	Once started a course, looks at progression from year 1-2, 2-3 etc and graduation. Up-dates history files
20	Educ_malcs	For males, processes exiting or continuing course	Once started a course, looks at progression from year 1-2, 2-3 etc and graduation. Up-dates history files
21	Educ_prim	Processes primary education	As function of age (in months) and state of residence
22	Educ_sect	Processes school sectors	Moves pupils between government, catholic and other sectors

23	Emig	Performs emigration	Computes probability of emigrating as function of sex, age, country of birth and marital status. Females over 17 and single males over 17 are randomly chosen to emigrate with their families. The crystal ball is up-dated accordingly.
24	General	A few ad hoc subroutines	For example: 'IN' returns true if a person is a member of the passed list; 'Ranuniom Table' – drand48(); 'RANUNI' returns ranuniom number from U[0,1] distribution; 'REL PRED' returns pointer to the predecessor of a person in the family
25	He_fns	Calculates hours worked and earnings	Calculates probability of people transiting – eg from working full time to part time or the other way round; or people not working to working, etc. Also computes the related changes in earnings
26	He_lgtfns	Functions relating to estimating hours/earnings	Box Cox transformation - $\log(x)$ or $\exp(y)$; normal distribution; months in employment; New Student; no labour experience; highest qualifications
27	Ind1prob	Probability re industry	Equations computing probability
28	Lfc_ctrl	Labour force calibration	Temporary tables created for the labour force calibration function
29	Lfc_qsort	Labour force calibration	Sorting procedure for the labour force calibrations. Has variou sorting routines plus printing first ten elements routines
30	Lfprob	Probabilities of a transition in the labour force	Logit equations for calculating the probability of a transition in the labour force (ie Employment, Unemployment, and Not in the Labour Force)
31	Lfupdt	Occupation, setor, industry routines	
33	Lgtfns	Last year's empl't situation	Months unemployed, in full time employment, etc
34	Llist	Bodnod maintenance	Routines relating to the maintenance of a bodnod linked list
35	Mstat		Updates marital status and records changes in status in history files
36	Occ1prob	Occupation probabilities	Equations defining probability of entering the various occupations

	Program	*sequencing*
37 **Main**	Establishes sequence for calling the above programs	While there is an 'overall' sequence of the programs called by Main, subroutines in various programs can be called outside that 'overall' pattern – eg when recalculating date of death following onset of disability. **Adjusted to allow consideration of variables by SES and to call the new program developed for the Health_SES and Health State Transition modules**
	Header files	
38 **Codes**	Lists all codes	For example Male (0), Female (1). **Adjusted to include the variable SES**
39 **Nodes**	Defines variables by structure	To the original list **we added the variables related to SES** .

NOTE: The programs in the original version of DYNAMOD that were modified for purposes of this thesis are indicated in **bold**.

Table A1.2: **List of key DYNAMOD variables**

Variable	Elements of variable
Sex	Male
	Female
Highest Qualification	Not yet at school
	At school
	Didn't finish secondary
	Completed Year 12
	Trade qualifications
	Diploma
	Bachelor degree
	Graduate diploma
	Masters degree
	Phd and higher qualifications
	Other
Study status	Full time
	Part time
Educational institution type	Government school
	Catholic school
	Other
	TAFE (Technical and Further Education)
	University – bachelors degree
	University – graduate diploma
	University - masters degree
	University – PhD or higher
Marital status	Never married
	Legally married
	Cohabiting
	Separated
	Divorced
	Widowed
Labour force status	Not in labour force
	Employee

	Employer
	Self employed
	Unemployed
	Unpaid labour
Employment status	Employed full time Employed part time, Self employed
	Not applicable
Country of birth	Australia
	Oceania
	UK or Ireland
	Southern EUROPE
	Other Europe and USSR
	Western Asia and Middle East
	Other Asia
	South America
	Other America
	Africa
	Other
Relationship in Family	Reference Person
	Spouse
	Dependent child
	Non-dependent child
	Other family
Hours worked per week	1_15
	16_24
	25_34
	35_39
	40
	41_48
	49 or more
Occupation	Managers
	Professionals and para-professionals
	Trade persons and clerks
	Sales persons

	Labourers
Industry	Agriculture
	Manufacturing
	Services
Employment sector	Government
	Private
State	NSW , VIC, QLD, SA, WA, TAS, NT, ACT
Immigrant type	Family reunion
	Skilled
	Independent
	Humanitarian
	Other visaed
	Non visaed
Type of dependent child	Natural or adopted child
	Step child of reference person
	Step child of a spouse
	Other child
Family's socioeconomic (SES) status	Most disadvantaged: SES quintile 1
	Least disadvantaged: SES quintile 5
Crystal ball events	Pre marital birth
	Marital birth
	Second & subsequent marital birth
	First Cohabitation
	Dissolution of first cohabitation
	Second and subsequent cohabitation
	Dissolution of 2nd and subseq. cohabs
	First marriage
	Dissolution of 1st marriage
	Cohabitation after marriage
	Second and subsequent marriage
	Dissolution of 2nd and subsequent marriage
	Divorce
	Pre marital pregnancy
	Marital pregnancy
	Second and subsequent marital pregnancy

	Date of Birth
	Data of Death
	Disable Date To
	Emigration

A1.2 The Wealth module

The Wealth module, which was subsequently added to DYNAMOD at the family level, is described in Kelly (2002; 2004). It accounts for the accumulation over the life course of five asset groups that make up a family's wealth: owner-occupied housing, superannuation, equities, rental investment properties and interest bearing deposits. Details on each asset group, based on Kelly (2002), are given below.

(a) Housing

Housing was found to be the biggest wealth asset of Australian families. Home ownership and the associated housing value and mortgage were imputed onto the starting population of DYNAMOD. The imputation was done on the basis of tenure, residential state, age and income.

(b) Superannuation

Superannuation was found to be the second most significant wealth asset. Two components were simulated, (i) the legislated compulsory component (the Superannuation Guarantee) which in 2002 amounted to 9% of earnings, and (ii) voluntary contributions distributed using probabilistic techniques to match aggregate ABS statistics.

In the model, the values of the assets grow in line with historical data and industry expectations for the future. At retirement, the funds are transferred to the individual's cash deposit account from where the model allows them to use these in the same way as other funds.

Thus the model allows people to save or dissave, depending on their total incomes, on historical expenditure patterns.

(c) Equities (shares)

ABS income survey data were used to impute the initial 1986 values of equities onto the model's base data. The values of equity assets were then updated in the simulation phase on an annual basis using actual and predicted changes to the 'All Ordinaries Price Index'.

(d) Rental properties

Although only around 6% of Australian families own a rental property, this asset was modeled because its value was quite high.

(e) Interest bearing cash deposits

Interest bearing cash deposits were found to be the most popular form of investment in Australia. The model simulates these as a savings residual after payments associated with other investments had been met. The interest earned is modeled as a lower rate for deposits up to A$5000 and a higher rate above that value.

A2 Possible data sources

Appendix A2 describes each of the data sources examined for possible use on this thesis. Chapter 3 draws on this Appendix when discussing the extent to which these sources meet the data requirements of the thesis (sections 3.1, 3.2 and 3.3). Chapter 3 also indicates which data sources have been chosen for use in the thesis (section 3.4).

Four data sources are described below: the Australia-wide National Health Surveys and Disability Surveys conducted by the ABS, the South Australian based Australian Longitudinal Study of Ageing and mortality statistics available from the AIHW. Because life course patterns are important in DYNAMOD, longitudinal data will be particularly important. However, it is generally acknowledged that, compared with other developed countries, Australia does not have a rich longitudinal database.[51] For this reason novel use was made of cross sectional data in this thesis (sections 8.1 and 8.3).

A2.1 National Health Surveys (1977, 1983, 1989 and 1995)

The 1995 National Health Survey (NHS) considered in this thesis was conducted by the Australian Bureau of Statistics (ABS) during the 12 months between January 1995 and January 1996. It involved Australia-wide interviews with some 23,800 non-institutionalised households (57,633 persons) (see ABS 1996a, p. 1). This sample comprised around one-third of one per cent of the Australian population.

The survey included:

---

[51] At the Forum on Research Study Design (1999) it was noted that, unlike many other developed countries, Australia had little data available through longitudinal surveys. It was also noted that the biggest benefits of longitudinal studies were their ability to establish *cause and effect* relationships (particularly lifetime relationships), to provide an indication of *emerging issues* and to indicate *transitions* (for example, in and out of disease states) – see section 3.1.

- a household questionnaire used for collecting basic demographic data (for example, sex, age, country of birth, occupation and relationship between individuals in each household); and

- a personal interview to obtain details on each individual about illnesses, health service and pharmaceutical usage and health related lifestyle issues.

Much of the health-related information in the 1995 survey is 'as reported' by respondents, and is not medically verified. This means that conditions that disrupt people's every day lives are more likely to have been reported accurately than conditions having only a minor effect. Also, respondents may have been reluctant to report certain medical conditions.

Nevertheless, drawing on international studies, the OECD concluded that perceived health status was a useful independent predictor of future health problems as well as mortality (OECD 1998, p.19).

The 1995 NHS survey also contained a supplementary survey which allows computation of the SF-36 physical and mental health scales (ABS 1996a, pp 149-51). The SF-36 survey included questions on Physical Functioning, Role-Physical, Bodily Pain, General Health, Vitality, Social Functioning, Role-Emotional and Mental Health. Some of these can lead to *'health transition indicators'* (eg items 11a, 11b and 11c, which are Sick Easier, As Healthy and Health to Get Worse).[52] Some of these were seen as possibly useful when deriving transition probabilities.

After further examination – see section 3.3 - we decided not to use the 1995 NHS in this thesis. This was because the National Health Surveys do not cover people living in institutions (eg nursing homes, hospitals, prisons, etc.). People in institutions comprise

---

[52] Hemingway et al 1997 found that the SF-36 was capable of detecting change in health in a general population.

a significant proportion of Australians aged 70 or over – a group of particular importance to this thesis.

A2.2 Australian Longitudinal Study of Ageing (ALSA)

The Australian Longitudinal Study of Ageing (ALSA) is Australia's first multi-dimensional population based study of ageing. It is the largest and most comprehensive study of persons aged over 70 years ever undertaken in Australia. The project is being conducted by the Centre for Ageing Studies, an affiliated research unit of the Flinders University of South Australia and a World Health Organization Collaborating Centre, based in Adelaide. The study brings together information on the health, social and economic circumstances of older persons.

The first round (Wave 1) of the ALSA began in September 1992. Information collected from 2,087 participants included a comprehensive personal interview, home based clinical assessments and self-completed questionnaires. A year later a brief telephone interview (Wave 2) was held with 1,779 available participants asking about any changes that had occurred. In September 1994 Wave 3 commenced with another extensive interview and assessment similar to Wave 1. 1,679 people participated in this round. Two more short telephone interviews followed in September 1995 (Wave 4) when 1,504 participants were interviewed. In February 1998 (Wave 5) 1,171 interviews were completed. Follow-up response rates have been about 90% or more. Beyond 1998 it was planned that a Wave 6 will take place with up to 1000 participants, involving comprehensive personal interviews, assessments and home visits.

All those in the study lived in the Adelaide metropolitan area and were originally chosen at random. Participants came from all walks of life and lived in many different situations: private homes, with family, in retirement villages and in nursing homes.

They included people in all categories of health with a wide range of functional abilities.

The ALSA was not chosen for use in this thesis because of its relatively small sample size and its focus on a capital city, rather than on all cities and country areas in Australia (section 3.2).

A2.3 Disability surveys

The Australian Bureau of Statistics (ABS) conducts disability surveys at five year intervals. Those already in the public domain are:

- 1981 Survey of Handicapped Persons;

- 1988 Survey of Disabled and Aged Persons;

- 1993 Survey of Disability, Ageing and Carers (ABS 1993b);

- 1998 Survey of Disability Ageing and Carers (ABS 1999b and c).

The 1993 and 1998 surveys used the definitions of disability and handicap as proposed by the World Health Organisation (WHO) in the International Classification of Impairments, Disabilities and Handicaps (ICIDH) 1980 - ABS (2002). For the forthcoming 2003 Survey the definitions of disability to be used will be as proposed by the WHO in the International Classification of Functioning, Disability and Health (ICF) 2001.

For this thesis we mainly used the 1998 survey – section 3.4. The sample for that survey included 15,715 private and special dwellings. The response rate was 93%. 37,580 persons were interviewed in households and 5,761 in cared accommodations. (ABS 1999b, p.13). Only 9% of the questionnaires were incomplete, due mainly to non-response to the question about the annual income of the family (section A6.2) – a family comprising the adults and dependent children whose income was shared within the household. In the unit record dataset used for purposes of this thesis – with just over 40,000 observations – the records with income-related non-responses were deleted. The completion rates for the questions on disability were close to 100%. Because respondents were interviewed in the dwellings they resided in, each questionnaire had the correct street address recorded on it by the trained ABS interviewer.

Although longitudinal analyses were not possible, the four surveys had much of their variables comparable (ABS 1999c, p.57). Thus we were able to study trends over time – section 9.2.

The World health Organisation (WHO) defines disability as "Any restriction or lack (resulting from an impairment) of ability to perform an activity in the manner or within the range considered normal for a human being." – ABS (2000a, p.3).

In the ABS's 1998 Survey *disability* is defined as a limitation, restriction or impairment, which has lasted, or is likely to last, for at least six months and restricts every day activities (ABS 1999c, p.66-7). The ABS notes that disability usually exists as a consequence of disease, disorder or injury – with physical conditions (such as musculoskeletal disorders) having been the most common cause (85% in 1998). However, mental or behavioural disorders were also significant (15% in 1998) – ABS 1999c, p.7.

A *long term health condition* is a disease or disorder, including damage from accidents or injuries, which has lasted, or is likely to last, for six months or more. Not all long term conditions restrict people in their everyday activities and result in a disability – ABS (2000a, p.3).

In relation to the effects of long term illness and disability ABS (2000a, p.3) notes that "There may be an effect on family ... and the wider community or an impact through reduced education or workforce participation. However, many people with disabilities and long term conditions are able to continue with their usual activities ... and others are enabled to do so with appropriate help. "

The *core activities* considered were communication, mobility and self care. Four levels of core activity *restrictions* were considered (ABS 1999c, p. 66):

- *mild*: needs no help and has no difficulty with any of the core activity tasks, but uses aids/equipment; or cannot easily walk 200 metres; or cannot walk up-down stairs without a handrail; or cannot easily bend to pick up an object from the floor; or cannot use public transport; or can use public transport but needs help/supervision; or needs no help/supervision but has difficulty with public transport;

- *moderate*: needs no help but has difficulty with a core activity task;

- *severe*: sometimes needs help with a core activity task; or has difficulty understanding or being understood by family or friends; or can communicate more easily using non-spoken forms of communication, such as sign language;

- *profound*: is unable to do, or always needs help with, a core activity task.

Compared with the National Health Surveys, the Disability Surveys conducted have the advantage of covering both households and institutions. The Disability Surveys thus provide a more complete picture of the health of the Australian population, especially of its older citizens aged 70 years or over.

The Disability Surveys are useful not only in indicating 'disability' status and severity, but also whether the respondent is restricted in schooling or employment activities and whether has long term health condition without disability. The 1998 survey also has questions on 'main disabling conditions' (close to 100 categories, based on ICD9 disease classifications which can be grouped into the priority areas of heart disease, cancer, diabetes, asthma, mental illness and injuries).

In the thesis we made use of the above mentioned levels of core activity restrictions –

Chapter 8 – and indicated that the data on 'main disabling conditions' could be used in

possible future extensions of the dynamic microsimulation model – section 13.2.

A2.4 Mortality statistics

A2.4.1 Causes of deaths (ABS)

Possible sources of data on Australians' health status are the 'causes of death'

publications by the ABS (1998a and earlier years). These data were examined because

they had the potential to provide a useful link between the date of death – as determined

in DYNAMOD - and the diseases underlying people's health status and disability status.

Also, the 'causes of death' data had the advantage over the self reported NHS data of

having been medically verified.

The 1998 ABS 'causes of death' statistics allow identification of the underlying cause

of death by ICD code (usually 3-digit ICD code), the number of causes reported, and the

relationship between multiple causes and the underlying cause.

While the 'causes of death' data were not used in the model building carried for this

thesis, their possible use in further model development– such as allocating key diseases

to individuals - was mentioned in section 13.2.

A2.4.2 Mortality by age sex and socioeconomic status

Special extracts by the Australian Institute of Health and Welfare (AIHW) were

obtained for this thesis from the AIHW's Mortality database. The extracts are by sex, 5-

year age groups, external and non-external causes of death and socioeconomic status -

as measured by quintiles of the ABS's index of 'Relative Socio-economic

Disadvantage' (Appendix A3). The most disadvantaged people are in quintile 1 and the least disadvantaged in quintile 5. The extract covers the 1995-97 period. The statistics in the AIHW's Mortality database were extensively used in Dunn et al (2002).

A3   Socio-economic indexes for areas (SEIFA)

The material presented in this Appendix is referred to in sections 2.1, 5.2 and A2.4.2.

The geographically-based Socioeconomic Indexes For Areas (SEIFA) used in this paper
were derived from the 1996 Census, based on the characteristics of the area of residence
of each census respondent (ABS 1998c). The smallest area for the indexes that are
available is the Census Collection District (CD). In urban areas a CD is roughly
equivalent to about 250 dwellings. In 1996 there were 34,500 CDs throughout Australia.

To cover different aspects of an area's socioeconomic conditions, the ABS developed
five types of indicators: Index of Relative Socio-Economic Disadvantage; Urban Index
of Relative Socio-Economic Advantage; Rural Index of Relative Socio-Economic
Advantage; Index of Education and Occupation and Index of Economic Resources. In
this paper, as in most studies of inequalities, the indicator of socioeconomic status used
was the Index of Relative Socio-Economic Disadvantage.

In developing the five types of SEIFA indexes, the ABS used the technique of Principal
Component Analysis. This is a multivariate method that summarises, for each CD, the
effects of a large number of area-related variables – such as educational qualifications;
employment status; occupation; family size; family income; housing (whether renting
from government or the private sector; or whether owning or purchasing dwellings);
number bedrooms per person; and car ownership. In essence, Principal Component
Analysis determines the 'weights' to be attached to the variables that make a significant
contribution to a particular index. For each type of SEIFA index, a different set of
variables were found to have significant weights. For example, for the Index of Relative
Socio-Economic Disadvantage the variables with the greatest weights were: low

income, low educational attainment, high unemployment and jobs in relatively unskilled occupations. For this index the variables measuring family wealth – such as home purchasing or ownership – had insignificant weights. By contrast, wealth-related variables had the greatest weights for the Index of Economic Resources.

With the Index of Relative Socio-Economic Disadvantage, those CDs that had a high proportion of residents with low income, low educational attainment, high unemployment and unskilled occupations, were classified into the lower SES quintiles. Conversely, those with a low proportion of such residents were classified into the higher SES quintiles.

The ABS cautions that the SEIFA indexes do not provide good measures for all social conditions. For example, it notes that the age structure of the population is not used directly in any of the indexes (ABS 1998c). This is of particular importance to studies of health inequalities because, as shown in the Results section of the main body of the text, age is the most important determinant of individuals' health status (as indicated by disability).

A4 Changes in mortality patterns by age and sex, 1990-92 to 1995-97

The material presented in this Appendix supports the findings described in section 6.2.1.

Considering mortality rates for all SES quintiles, the patterns for the 1995-97 period were very similar to those embedded in the original DYNAMOD *input data* – which used data for the period 1990-92. This is shown in Figure A4.1 for all cause mortality and Figure A4.2 for non-external causes – that is for the disabled. The figures were charted after the AIHW data by 5-year age groups were smoothed to produce rates for single years of age (section 6.2.1).

Distinction between the genders was found to be important. Figure A4.1 indicates that, in both time periods and for most age groups, all cause mortality rates were significantly lower for women than for men. Although not charted, the differences across quintiles were also found to be significantly smaller for women than for men.

Both Figures indicate a decline in mortality rates in the 1995-97 period compared with the 1990-92 period, with the trend being considerably stronger for mortality arising from non-external causes. This is in line with the findings of a French study that mortality rates by age declined significantly between 1985-87 and 1995-97 (Robine, 2001). It is interesting to note that in the French study, where data was available by single years of age, a decline in mortality rate occurred for each single year of age. The pattern was similar with the Australian data at the 5-year age group level. The occasional reversal of this trend in the charts below arises from the smoothing process we applied to the original AIHW data (required for input data to DYNAMOD).

Figure A4.1: **Mortality rates, all causes, by age and sex, 1990-92 and 1995-97**

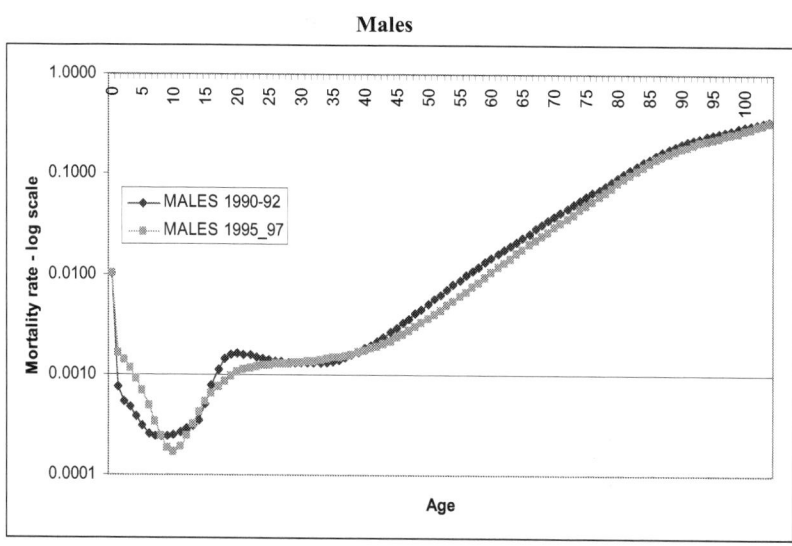

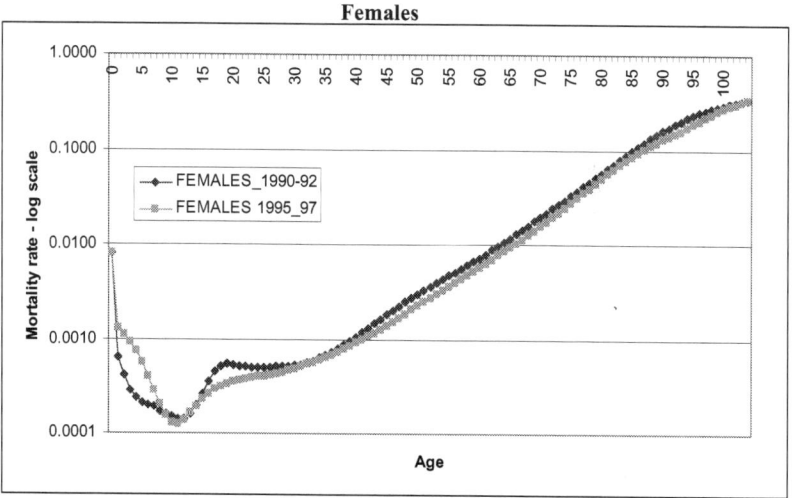

Sources: input data to DYNAMOD - ABS (1993a) and computations for this thesis using the AIHW extract, 1995-97.

Figure A4.2: **Mortality rates, non-external causes (ie the disabled population), by age and sex, 1990-92 and 1995-97**

Males

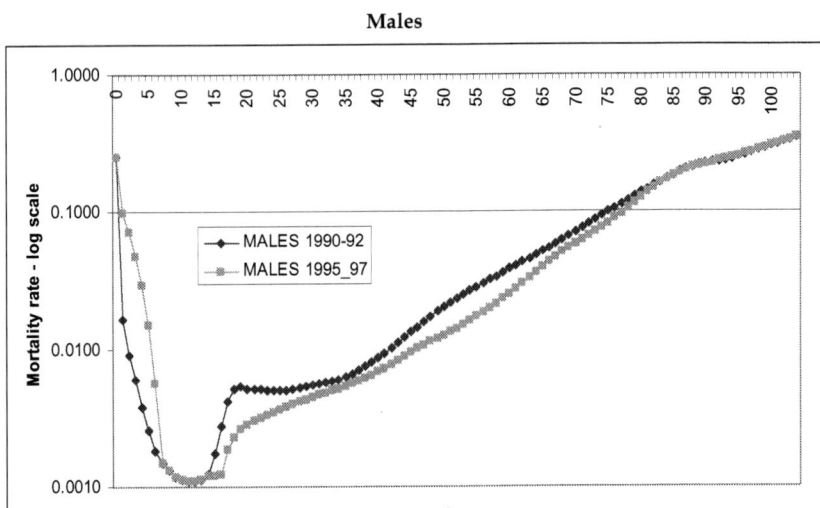

Females

Sources: input data to DYNAMOD - ABS (1993a) and computations for this thesis using the AIHW extract, 1995-97.

Figure A4.3 charts the AIHW data by 5-year age groups for all cause mortality by age, sex and SEIFA quintiles. It shows that differences in mortality rates across SES quintiles were greater for men than women, and that - across all age groups - all cause mortality rates were higher for men than for women.

Figure A4.3: **Mortality rates, all causes by age and SEIFA quintiles, 1995-7**

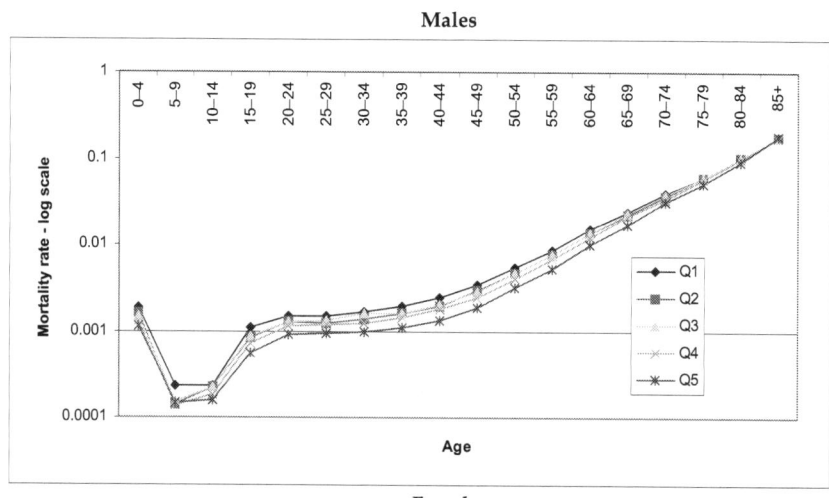

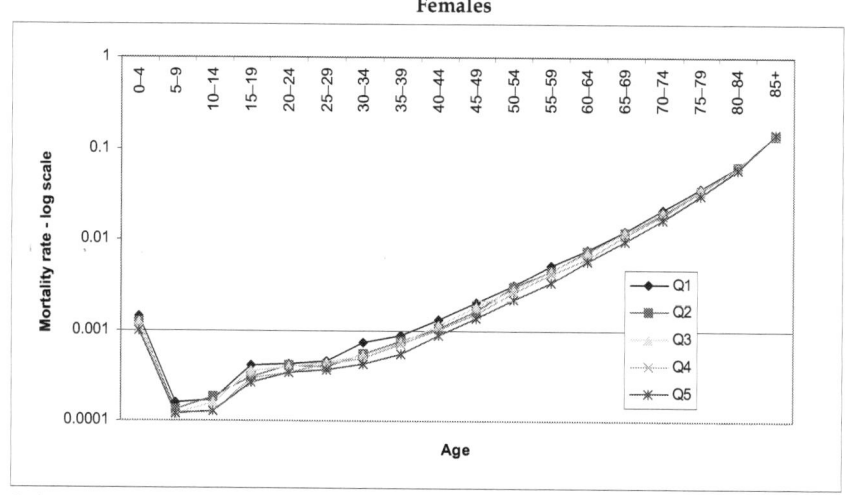

Q1 is most disadvantaged and Q5 the least disadvantaged quintile.
Sources: computations for this thesis using AIHW mortality data extract. SEIFA quintile 1

A5 Changes in disability prevalence by age and sex, 1993 and 1998

The material presented in this Appendix supports the findings described in section 6.3.

Figure A5.1 charts, for all SES quintiles, the proportion of the disabled by single years

of age for 1993 and 1998.

Figure A5.1: **Disability rates by age and sex, 1993 and 1998**

Males

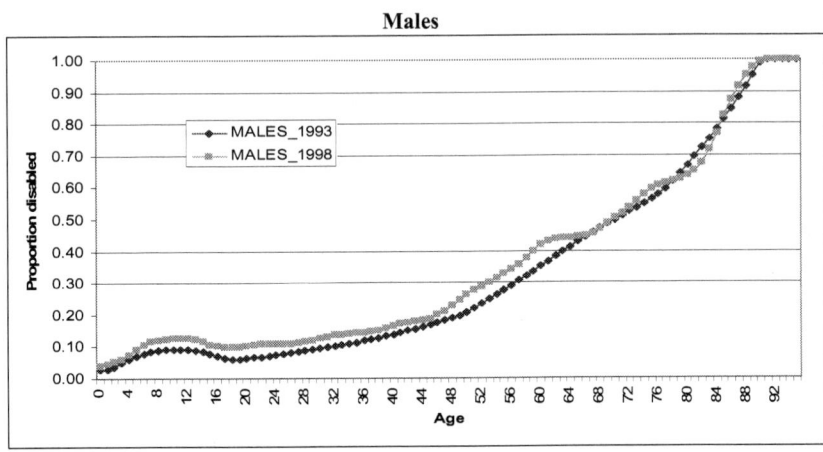

Females

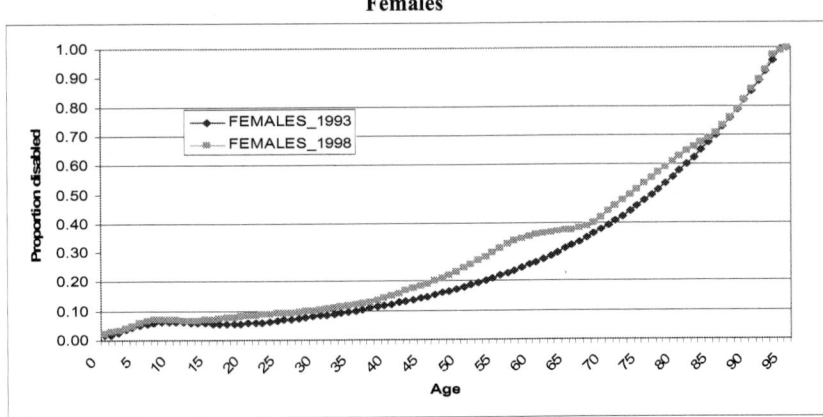

Sources: Disability surveys (ABS 1993c and 1999a). Note that in these surveys years of age above 85 are available as a single 85+ grouping.

A striking feature of the charts is the steady and accelerating increases in disability rates from age 40 onwards. By age 80 years, around 60% of men and 50% of women have become 'disabled' - based on the definitions in the ABS's disability surveys. Another noteworthy feature is that the onset of disability occurs at younger ages for men than for women.

Figure A5.1 also suggests that disability rates increased between 1993 and 1998. However, as seen in Chapter 9 (section 9.2), this may to some extent be due to differences in the way the two Disability surveys having been conducted – see section 6.3.

A6 Deriving income-based SES indicators from the 1998 Disability Survey

This Appendix describes the way income-based SES indicators were constructed from the 1998 Disability survey (ABS 1999a) when developing the disability related input data by socioeconomic status – required for the new Health_SES and Health State Transition modules. It supports the material presented in sections 3.4, 4.3, and 5.2.

There is considerable debate in the literature as to how to interpret income data from ABS and other surveys when searching for a proxy for socioeconomic disadvantage. Issues include whether it is more appropriate to use expenditure rather than income data; whether 'self declared' income information can be considered accurate; whether to consider weekly or annual income; whether after tax, rather than gross income would be more appropriate; and whether adjustments should be made for government transfers, such as unemployment benefits, the age pension, etc.

For this thesis we used the same data source for income as for disability, that is the ABS's 1998 Disability survey. While this has the important advantage of being able to obtain *both* the income and disability information for the same individual or family, it also has limitations. For example expenditure information is not available from the Disability survey.

Re accounting for government taxes and transfers, we did not consider these when preparing the enhanced model's Base data. However, in its simulation years DYNAMOD computes both taxes and transfers, so by the first year of interest to this thesis, that is 1998, the income information we used did account for government taxes and transfers.

Analyses using the Disability survey prior to the results entering DYNAMOD were carried out using the SAS programming language. The related code can be made available on request.

In this Appendix we first describe how a SAS compatible dataset was constructed from the ABS's unit record data files (ABS 1999a), so that individuals' characteristics could be linked to their family level characteristics - such as family income and size (section A6.1). Then we describe the processes used for computing family income – and, from these, family income quintiles (section A6.2).

A6.1 Creating the basic SAS dataset

The 1998 Disability Survey unit record files are made available by the ABS as separate datasets at the levels of:

- household;

- family;

- income unit;

- person;

- disability;

- primary carer;

- carer.

The ABS also provided a 'Formats' folder with the above dataset, facilitating the identification of the many variables provided, but making the installation and the use of the data more complicated than with most earlier ABS unit record datasets.

In this thesis we needed variables available in the first five datasets. Because the analyses carried out required variables from any of these, it was necessary to find linkages across the datasets so that variables relating to a particular person could be brought together, regardless of the dataset they had been originally included in. For example, the equivalent income variable (at income unit, or 'iu', level) needed to be computed using the 'iu' income and 'iu' size ABS variables, and then the new equivalent income variable (computed for the thesis) had to be brought across to the Person dataset. In addition, the equivalent 'iu' income had to be applied to each 'iu' member, since all members of an income unit have a common 'family' income.

For purposes of this Appendix, the linking of individuals across these different datasets is illustrated by the following example. Putting the original ABS variables in between 'quotes', the following identification (ID) numbers were generated, starting with the highest level of aggregation (that is the Household):

hh_id = 'id402'

fam_id = 10*'id402' + 'id408'

iu_id = 100*'id402' + 10*'id408' +'id409'

pers-id = 1000*id402 + 100*'id408' + '10*'id409' + 'id410'

With: 'id402'   being the ABS person level random ID in the Person dataset;

'id408'   being the family number (person level) in the Person dataset;

'id409'   being the income unit number (person level) in the Person dataset; and

'id410'   being the person number (within 'iu') in the Person dataset.

Similar ID numbers were constructed within the other datasets of relevance to this thesis, with the Disability ID numbers being arrived at in the same way (since the Disability dataset is at the person level), and a lesser number of ID being generated for the other datasets (ie three for the 'iu' dataset at household, family and 'iu' levels and only one in the household dataset, at the household level).

Once these coherent ID-s had been computed, it was possible to merge variables across the five datasets, using the relevant ID as 'by' variable in the MERGE command of the SAS programming language.

A6.2 Deriving family income and computing income quintiles

As noted in section 5.2, income was one of the variables used to indicate socioeconomic status in this thesis. We computed income quintiles at the family level using the 'Total weekly cash income' variable in the 'income unit' file of the 1998 Disability survey. This variable is presented in groupings of 'no income', 'less than $80' and then at $40 intervals to $1159, with '$1160 or over' being the last income category. 'Refusal' or 'don't know' responses accounted for 9.6 per cent of income units.

First, assuming random distribution within groupings, a dollar value for income was allocated to families within each income group. Next, the 'family income' and 'equivalent family income' variables were computed for each family, as defined in section 5.2.[53] Finally, the Australian population was divided into five equal groups – ie quintiles - by the 'family income' or 'equivalent family income' variable, and an indicator was attached to each family as to which of the five quintiles they belonged to. Because the same SES quintile was allocated to each family member, children and non-working spouses – who initially had no income recorded in the Disability survey – were classified into the same quintile as their family as a whole.

Next the desired variables from the household and person files of the 1998 Disability Survey were merged with the above modified 'income unit file'. Also, the records with

---

[53] Note that the term 'family' has been used throughout the Chapters of this thesis as being a proxy for the ABS's 'income unit' concept. ABS (2003, Appendix 1) defines 'income unit' as adults and dependent children within a household whose income is shared.

non-responses (re income) - ie 9.6 per cent of income units - were deleted, the resulting

dataset containing just over 40,000 person records. An alternative would have been to

allocate an income to the 'non-response' group in proportion to the overall income

distribution indicated by the records with responses. However, this option would have

distorted the disability (and other non-income) characteristics of the population by

income quintile. Noting that the distributions of the 'responding' and 'total' populations

by age - one of the key determinants of both health and SES – only differed from

between -1% and +2% across each of the broad age groups (0-19, 20-39, 40-59, 60-69

and 70+), we concluded that the bias arising from deletion of the 9.6% of income units

with 'non-response' was likely to be small.

Given the importance of disability to our analyses, and the small bias expected to arise

from deletion of the records with income non-response, we chose the 'deletion' option.

A6.3 Example of SAS code: deriving income-based SES indicators

This section provides the SAS code for the material described in sections A6.1 and

A6.2.

```
Data tp1;
Set data98cd.dsb98psn;    /* sets ABS Disab98 Survey 'person' dataset */

        wtp=WT401/10000;                        /* person level weight */
        hh_id=id402;
        fam_id=id402*10+id408;
        iu_id=id402*100+id408*10+id409;
        pers_id=id402*1000+id408*100+id409*10+id410;
Run;

PROC SORT DATA=tp1;
        BY iu_id;

PROC FREQ DATA=tp1;
        TABLES INC400;                          /* person level income */
        WEIGHT wtp;
    Run;

    Data tp2;
    Set data98cd.dsb98unt;   /* Disability98 Survey 'inc unit' dataset */
            wtp_iu=WT301/10000;                 /* h'hold weight (iu level)
*/
            x = RANUNI(987654321);          /* random No between 0 and 1 */
```

```
        hh_id=id302;
        fam_id=id302*10+id308;
        iu_id=id302*100+id308*10+id309;

        /* total weekly cash income (iu level) */
/* generate dollar values from bracket incomes */

        If inc300 GT 29 then inc_iu=9999;
            else if inc300=00 then inc_iu = 0;
            else if inc300=01 then inc_iu = 10 + (80-10)* x;
            else if inc300=02 then inc_iu = 80 + (119-80)* x;
            else if inc300=03 then inc_iu = 120 + (159-120)* x;
            else if inc300=04 then inc_iu = 160 + (199-160)* x;
            else if inc300=05 then inc_iu = 200 + (239-200)* x;
            else if inc300=06 then inc_iu = 240 + (279-240)* x;
            else if inc300=07 then inc_iu = 280 + (319-280)* x;
            else if inc300=08 then inc_iu = 320 + (359-320)* x;
            else if inc300=09 then inc_iu = 360 + (399-360)* x;
            else if inc300=10 then inc_iu = 400 + (439-400)* x;
            else if inc300=11 then inc_iu = 440 + (479-440)* x;
            else if inc300=12 then inc_iu = 480 + (519-480)* x;
            else if inc300=13 then inc_iu = 520 + (559-520)* x;
            else if inc300=14 then inc_iu = 560 + (599-560)* x;
            else if inc300=15 then inc_iu = 600 + (639-600)* x;
            else if inc300=16 then inc_iu = 640 + (679-640)* x;
            else if inc300=17 then inc_iu = 680 + (719-680)* x;
            else if inc300=18 then inc_iu = 720 + (759-720)* x;
            else if inc300=19 then inc_iu = 760 + (799-760)* x;
            else if inc300=20 then inc_iu = 800 + (839-800)* x;
            else if inc300=21 then inc_iu = 840 + (879-840)* x;
            else if inc300=22 then inc_iu = 880 + (919-880)* x;
            else if inc300=23 then inc_iu = 920 + (959-920)* x;
            else if inc300=24 then inc_iu = 960 + (999-960)* x;
            else if inc300=25 then inc_iu = 1000 + (1039-1000)* x;
            else if inc300=26 then inc_iu = 1040 + (1079-1040)* x;
            else if inc300=27 then inc_iu = 1080 + (1119-1080)* x;
            else if inc300=28 then inc_iu = 1120 + (1159-1120)* x;
            else if inc300=29 then inc_iu = 1160 + (2000-1160)* x;

        If IU310 in ('0','1') then fam_size=1;

/* set up family size variable */
            else if IU310='2' then fam_size=2;
            else if IU310='3' then fam_size=3;
            else if IU310='4' then fam_size=4;
            else if IU310='5' then fam_size=5;
            else if IU310 IN ('6','7') then fam_size=6;

/* computes equivalence factor (iui level) */

        If IU300='1' and fam_size=2 then FACTOR=(1+0.5);
            else if IU300='2' then FACTOR= (1+0.5) +(fam_size-2)*0.3;
            else if IU300='3' then FACTOR= 1 +(fam_size-1)*0.3;
            else if IU300 in ('0','4') then FACTOR = 1;

/* identifies income non-responses (iu level) */
/* computes equivalent family income variable (iu level) */

if inc_iu=9999 then eq_inc_iu=9999;
        else if inc_iu NE 9999 then eq_inc_iu=inc_iu/FACTOR;

/* deletes records with income non-response */

if inc_iu=9999 then delete;
```

```
Run;

PROC SORT DATA=tp2;
     BY iu_id;

Data tp3;
Set data98cd.dsb98hsh;          /* household level dataset */
   wtp_hsh=WT101/10000;
   hh_id=id102;

   if HSH120=0 then dis_hhd=0;
      else if HSH120=1 then dis_hhd=1;
      else if HSH120 in (2,3) then dis_hhd=2;
Run;

PROC SORT DATA=tp3;
     BY hh_id;

/* obtains Disab98 person level dataset with hhold variables added */

Data hhold_merge;
     merge tp1 tp3;
       by hh_id;
 Run;

PROC SORT DATA=hhold_merge;
     BY iu_id;

PROC FREQ DATA=tp2;
   TABLES INC300;
   WEIGHT wtp_iu;
 Run;
```

Next, a SAS macro program is then called to compute quintiles of equivalent family income.

A7 Demographic, health, employment and residential characteristics of Australians, 1998

A7.1 Introduction

Using the 1998 Disability survey, in this Appendix the demographic, employment and residential (ie whether living in households or institutions) characteristics of Australians are examined as a function of their disability/illness status. When relevant, the population groups by the four health states defined in Chapter 8 (section 8.2) are used.

Findings reported in this Appendix are referred to in the main body of the text in sections 3.3, 4.3, 8.1, 12.3 and 13.2.

A7.2 Disability by age and sex

As shown in Chapters 4 and 8 (sections 4.3 and 8.1), age was a main factor influencing the prevalence of disability in 1998. While up to age 30 only about 10 per cent of the population had a disability, by age 80 that proportion had risen to above 60 per cent. As for 1993 – see Antcliff et al 1996, Fig A1, p. 104 – the 1998 data indicated that, for most age groups, the disability rate was slightly higher for males than for females.

Figures A7.2.1 and A7.2.2 show that, up to age 40, a lower proportion of women had a severe disability than men.

The proportions were similar for both sexes in the 40 to 70 age group, however over age 70 a higher proportion of women had severe disability than men. A possible explanation for these patterns is that women tend to live longer. Thus women are likely to reach the 'severe disability' stage later in life than men.

Figure A7.2.1: **Proportion of Males by age group and disability level, 1998**

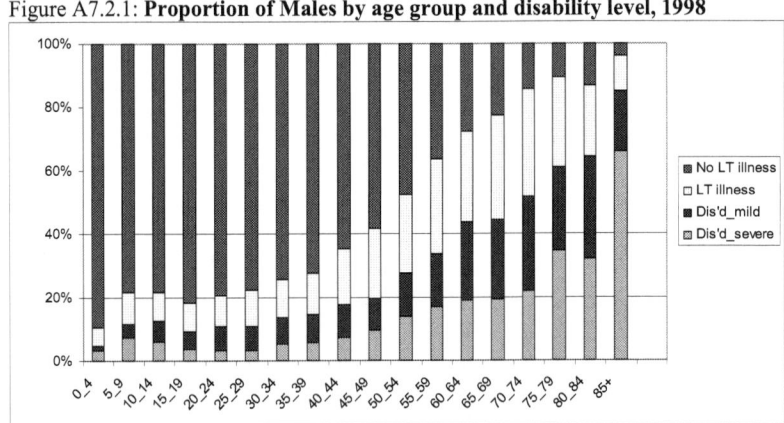

Source: 1998 Disability Survey (ABS 1999a).

Figure A7.2.2: **Proportion of Females by age group and disability level, 1998**

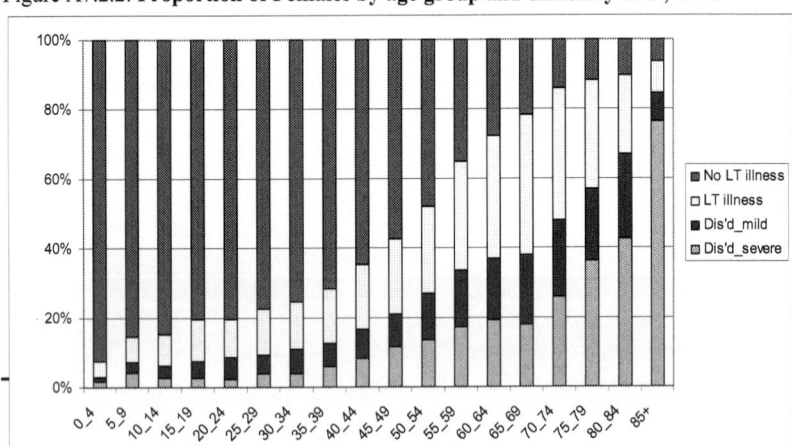

Source: 1998 Disability Survey (ABS 1999a)

The pattern was similar for mild disability, but generally a higher proportion of women had long term illness than men. With regard to 'no long term illness', a significantly higher proportion of women were disease or accident free up to the age of 25, but beyond that age there did not seem to be much difference between the sexes.

The above figures have been referred to in sections 3.3 and 8.1.

A7.3 The disabled population by income

Figure A7.3.1 shows that a much higher proportion of people were disabled in the two

lowest quintiles (the less well off group) than in the top three quintiles (the better off

group).

Figure A7.3.1: **Proportion of population disabled (mild and severe), by equivalent income quintile, 1998**

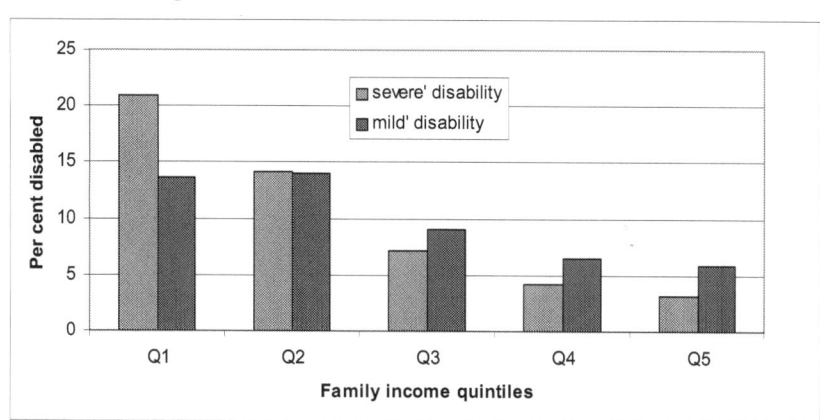

Source: 1998 Disability Survey (ABS 1999a). NOTE: Quintiles are equivalent income quintiles (income unit level) – Quintile 1 is the most disadvantaged and Quintile 5 the least disadvantaged.

In addition, this disability 'gap' between better off and the less well off Australians was

particular pronounced amongst people with severe disabilities. Also, while a greater

proportion of the less well off had severe disabilities than mild disabilities, this pattern

was reversed for the better off group (ie a lower proportion had severe disabilities than

mild disabilities).

Regarding the able-bodied, additional analyses showed that a significantly lower

proportion of the poorer group were free of long term conditions than the better off

group (around half compared with 70 per cent). However, the proportions with at least

one long term condition did not vary much across income quintiles.

The patterns reported in this section were referred to in section 4.3.

A7.4 The disabled population by labour force status and institutionalisation

Table A7.4.1 shows that those not disabled were much more likely to be employed than the disabled. While 46% of Australians aged 15 years or more were employed in 1998, with 27% 'not in the labour force' (NILF), amongst the severely disabled in that age group only 19.7% were employed, with 66.1% NILF. Also, those with long term illness or severe disability tended not to enter the labour force (37 to 66 per cent compared with 16 per cent for the healthiest group), rather than being classified as unemployed (3.9 to 2.7 per cent compared with 4.7 per cent for the healthiest group).

Table A7.4.1: **Proportion of persons aged 15 years or more by health and labour force status, 1998** (per cent)

Disability status	Empl'd	Unempl'd	NILF**	na*	Total
Disabled_severe	19.7	2.7	66.1	11.5	100
Disabled_mild	40.5	5.2	53.9	0.4	100
long term illness	49.7	3.9	36.7	9.7	100
No disab or LT illness	51.3	4.7	15.6	28.4	100
All Australians	46.3	4.4	27.1	22.2	100

Source: 1998 Disability Survey (ABS 1999a),. * not applicable- incl. persons in institutions; ** not in the labour force.

The patterns in table A7.4.1 were referred to in section 4.3.

Table A7.4.2 shows that very few Australians lived in institutions (just over 2% in 'health establishments' and 'other special dwellings'), with the vast majority residing in private dwellings. Nearly all people in 'health establishments' were severely disabled, while over half of people in 'other special dwellings' had neither long term illness nor disability.

Table A7.4.2: **Proportion of total population in private dwellings and institutions, 1998** (per cent)

	Severely disabled	Mild or no disability	Long term illness	No disab or illness	Total
Private dwelling	8.82	9.79	16.71	62.38	97.70
Health establish't	1.06	0.04	0.02	0.01	1.13
Other dwelling	0.20	0.15	0.28	0.55	1.18
All Australians	10.07	9.98	17.01	62.94	100

Source: 1998 Disability Survey (ABS 1999a).

The patterns in table 7.4.2 were referred to in section 3.3.

A7.5 Duration of main disabling condition and patterns of comorbidities

Figure A7.5.1 charts the proportions of the population, with 'main disabling conditions' recorded, within 'duration' groupings. It indicates that the majority of the disabled had the main condition causing their disability for less than 15 years.

An exponential trend line was fitted to the pattern in Figure 7.5.1 (R square 0.996), and could be used to project population shares for durations greater than 40 years. The trend equation could also be used to allocate 'single year of duration' to the 35% of Australians for whom a duration statistic was recorded in the 1998 survey. The equation could also be used to determine the incidence of disability - ie, for each person in the survey, by subtracting 'duration' from that person's age (after having converted the 5-year age groups of the survey to single years of age).

Figure A7.5.1: **Proportion of the population by duration of main disabling condition, 1998**

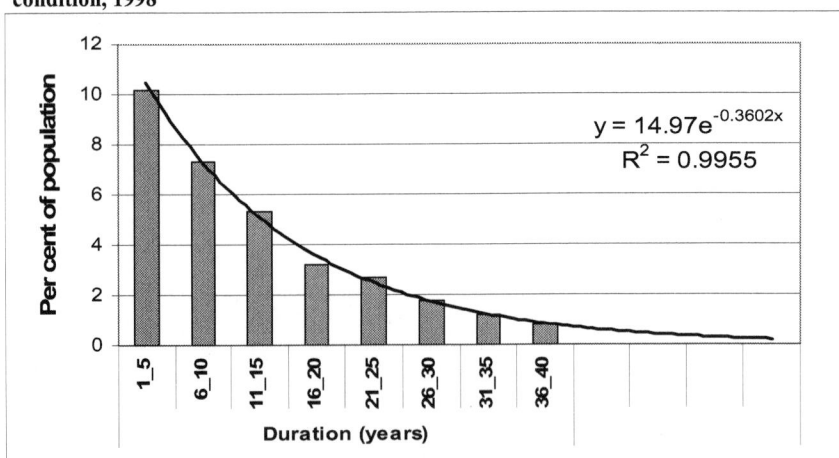

Source: 1998 Disability Survey (ABS 1999a), using the 'how long since main disabling condition occurred' variable.

Figure A7.5.2 shows that close to 18 per cent of the population had one health condition, with just over 8 per cent with two conditions. The 180 or so health conditions covered in the 1998 Disability survey range from blackouts, fainting, shortness of breath, glaucoma … to the main 'killer' diseases, such as cancers and cardiovascular disease.

Overall, while modelling comorbidities seems desirable, the patterns in Figures A7.5.1 and A7.5.2 suggest that focus on one condition per person – such as the 'main disabling condition' - could be satisfactory as an initial step.

Figure A7.5.2: **Proportion of population with one, two …nine conditions, 1998**

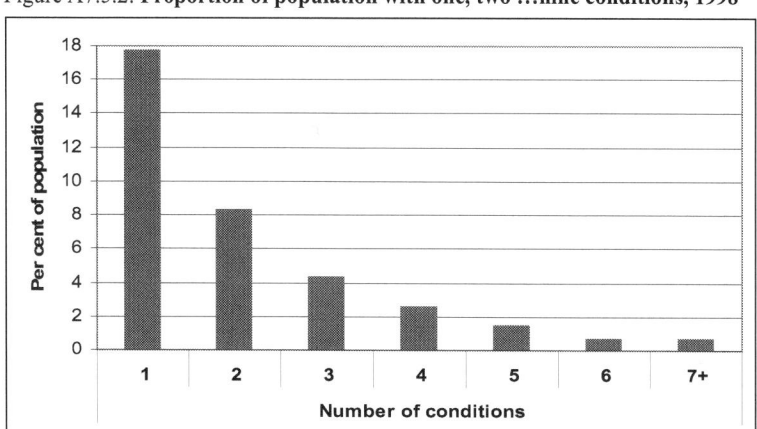

Source: 1998 Disability Survey (ABS 1999a).

The findings in this section have not been used in the model building part of the thesis. However, they were referred to in section 13.2 as being of potential use in possible future work.

A8   The modified OECD equivalence scale

Equivalent family income is a measure of income adjusted for the differing needs of various families (eg due to differences in family size). The aim is to have a measure through which the economic resources – and thus the standard of living - of different families can be compared. For further detail see Saunders (1996, pp 115-8).

In DYNAMOD, once the gross incomes (earned and/or received from government) of adults in the family had been added up to obtain the family's income, equivalent family income was computed using the modified OECD scale (Mejer and Siermann, 2000). This method uses equivalence scale factors (ESF) with:

-       a weight of 1 for the first adult in the family;

-       a weight of 0.5 for each subsequent adult in the family; and

-       a weight of 0.3 for each dependent child.

The equation for the equivalent family income (EFI) is:

EFI = Gross Family Income/ESF

These family-based EFI values were then assigned to each family member.

This Appendix was referred to in sections 5.2 and 7.2 of the main body of the text.

A9 Health as a reason for not looking for work

We used the 1998 Disability survey (ABS 1999a) to study the reasons given by respondents without a job as to why they were not looking for work. Amongst the six available responses two related to health: 'own health' and 'ill health/disability other than self'. We disaggregated the data by age, so as to gain an insight into differences in the reasons given between the younger and older age groups.

Because 88% of the 65-69 age group gave the 'retired' or 'too old' reason, that survey could not be used for establishing the importance of health amongst the reasons why 65-70 year olds were not looking for work. Table A9.1 summarises the findings for 25 to 64 year olds.

Table A9.1: **Main reason as to why not looking for work, by age, 1998**

Type of reason	Men			Women		
Age	*25-44*	*45-54*	*55-64*	*25-44*	*45-54*	*55-64*
1:'retired' or 'too old'*	3	5	54	1	13	59
2: own ill health/disability	48	77	39	9	25	17
3: study	31	3	1	7	3	0
4: does not need/want to work	4	4	1	7	25	12
5: ill health/disability other than self	1	1	1	6	12	5
6: all other reasons	13	11	4	71	22	8
Total	100	100	100	100	100	100

Source: 1998 Disability Survey, unit record files (ABS 1999a).

The main reason for not looking for work amongst 25-44 year olds was 'own health' for men (48%) and 'other reasons' for women (71%). For 45-54 year olds, 'own health' became much more important (77% for men and 25% for women). Also, around a quarter of women in that age group gave 'don't need/want to work' as the main reason. For both men and women aged 55-64 years, the main reason stated was 'retired/too old' (54% and 59% respectively). This suggests that ill health, although it may have been important had work been seen as a possibility, was not the reason recorded.

This Appendix was referred to in section 12.3.2.

A10 Age standardisation across SES quintiles

As seen in section 5.5.2 (Table 3), age is a considerably more important factor explaining disability than SES or sex. Thus, when analysing inequalities in the proportion disabled across quintile 'totals' between quintile 1 and quintile 5 populations – as in Table 2, section 5.5.1 - it is important to adjust for the effects of the differences that exist in the age distributions of SES quintiles. Without such adjustment, the differences in the Q1/Q5 disability rate ratios in the 'Totals' rows of Table 2 would be mainly due to 'age effects' - thus masking the effects due to SES effects, which is what Table 2 is attempting to measure.

The usual way of eliminating the effects of age differences across populations is to use the technique of age standardisation. This initially involves selecting a *standard population* with a fixed age structure. The disability rate for any other population is then adjusted to allow for discrepancies in age structures between the standard population and the population under study.

In this thesis the direct method of age standardisation is used, as set out in Armitage and Berry (1994, pp. 436–9). We chose the 1998 Australian population by age and SEIFA quintile as the *standard population* (estimated from ABS 1999a) ensured that the standardisation process eliminated the effect of age in the Q1/Q5 estimates (Table 2). Using this method, the age-standardised mean (or average) proportion disabled in a given SEIFA quintile population is:

$$\overline{X}_{as} = \frac{\sum\limits_{i} N_i \overline{x}_i}{\sum\limits_{i} N_i}$$

where :

$\overline{X}_{as}$ is the age-standardised mean;

N_i is the size of the *standard population* in the SEIFA quintile for age group i; and

$\overline{x}_i$ is the original proportion disabled for the SEIFA quintile population under study for age group i.

Overall, age standardisation produces an estimate of the mean that would have prevailed in the *standard population* of the SEIFA quintile under consideration if it had experienced the original age specific 'proportions disabled' within Q1 and Q5 (as indicated in the two middle columns of Table 2).

A11 Standard errors and statistical significance

Statistical testing for significance regarding the difference (or ratio) between

'proportions disabled' computed for two situations was carried out through the z-test

generally used in the literature (Mathers 1994, p.5). Assuming a normal distribution:

$$z = \frac{\text{Difference in the two proportions}}{\text{Standard error of the difference}}$$

At the 95 per cent level (for a one-tailed test), the two proportions – over age groups -

are significantly different if the calculated z exceeds 1.645. If $\overline{X}_1$ and $\overline{X}_2$ are the two

proportions and $SE(\overline{X}_1)$ and $SE(\overline{X}_2)$ their standard errors then are:

$$z = \frac{(\overline{X}_1 - \overline{X}_2)}{\sqrt{SE_1^2(\overline{X}_1) + SE_2^2(\overline{X}_2)}}$$

A12 Example of C code – computing and imputing socio-economic status

The algorithms for computing various forms of family level socioeconomic status in the model were described in section 7.2. The numerous cross-linkages needed with the original C code to obtain the required income, family size and wealth variables were described in Appendix A1 (Table A1.1).

As an example of the extensive C programming undertaken for this thesis, below is an extract of the C code used to compute and impute the various SES indicators:

```
/* Description of SES module:

 Computes each January the equivalent income/wealth SES indicator
for the previous year, as well as SES quintiles. Returns this as the SES_index
variable (0-4, 0 being the most disadvantaged). Attaches SES_index to each
DYNAMOD family (the same index to each family member)

*/

/********************* Defines           ***************************/

#define YearlyReturn 0.052

#define AGEGRPS   8    /* 0-14 15-24 25-34 35-44 45-54 55-64 65-74 75+ */

#define age_0014  0
#define age_1524  1
#define age_2534  2
#define age_3544  3
#define age_4554  4
#define age_5564  5
```

```
#define age_6574  6
#define age_75    7
```

```
/******************** Variables        ***************************/
```

```
extern short NOW;
```

```
extern int SES_index;  /* SES quintile of the person's family at current time */
```

```
extern int birth_SES_index;  /* SES quintile of the person's family at birth */
```

```
extern int health;         /* health status of individuals */
```

```
extern DTable *world[];
```

```
long heads [MAXPOP];
```

```
int   nkids_SES     ( Dynanode *dn); /* used when computing family size */
```

```
/******************** Prototypes       ***************************/
```

```
void SM_SES ( void );
```

```
int compare(void *, void *);
```

```
double betw (double a, double x, double y);
```

```
//******************************************************************
/******************** DD SEstatus      ***************************/
/* DESC:
```

Function computes combined income-wealth indicator of socioeconomic

status. SES_status is a continuous indicator, which is then transformed into a

quintile (0-4), ie the SES_index.

```
*/
```

```
void SM_SES ( void )
{
      Dynanode *dn,
       *sp,
      *head,
       *kid;
```

```
long        taxinc_r,       /* taxable income of family head that year */
            transinc_r,     /* transfer income of family head that year */
            taxinc_s,       /* taxable income of spouse that year */
            transinc_s,     /* transfer income of spouse that year */

            totwealth_f,    /* family's wealth (allocated to the family head) */
            YrWorth_f,      /* family's SE indicator in year */

            CutOff0,        /* cut-off value of SES_status for quintile 0 */
            CutOff1,        /* cut-off value of SES_status for quintile 1 */
            CutOff2,        /* cut-off value of SES_status for quintile 2 */
            CutOff3;        /* cut-off value of SES_status for quintile 3 */

int         TotPop,         /* persons in the total population at that time */
            QuintSize,      /* the number of persons in each SES quintile */

            CURRYEAR,       /* current year */
            nkids,          /* number of dependent children */
            NumFam,         /* number of persons in family */
            age,
            n,
            a,
            SES_index55,
            SES1,
            SES2,
            SES3,
            SES4,
            SES5,
            Dep,
            sex,
double      Factor, /* for computing equivalent family SES */
            i,
            j,
            k,
int         quintile;
int         AgeGrp;


//********************************************************************
//            Compute family's SES indicator
//
//********************************************************************
```

```
if (NOW > 1159)   /* start computations in 1987 */
{
        CURRYEAR = (NOW - 1159)/12 + 1986;

        dn = wctrl_first(world);              /* go to first person in population */
        printf("\nStarting SE Status Computation\n");

   do
   {

        if (dn->relpos == FP_REF)
        {
                sp = dn->spouse[LV];

                taxinc_r = dn->my.taxinc;

                transinc_r = dn->my.transinc;

                totwealth_f = dn->my.totwealth;

                    nkids= 0;

                    head = dn;

                    kid = dn;

                do
                {
                if ((kid->relpos) == FP_DEP_CHILD)
                        {
                        nkids++;
                        }
                } while ((kid=kid->rel) != head);


                if (sp != NULL)   /* computations when there is a spouse */
        {
                        taxinc_s = sp->my.taxinc;

                        transinc_s = sp->my.transinc;

                        NumFam = nkids + 2;

                        Factor = 1 + 0.5 + nkids*0.3;
```

```
        }

   else if (sp == NULL)    /* computations when there is no spouse */
      {
                  taxinc_s = 0;

                  NumFam = nkids + 1;

                  Factor = 1 + nkids*0.3;

      }

/* compute family's total income and total income_wealth */

        dn-> TotFamInc=(taxinc_r + taxinc_s) + (transinc_r+transinc_s);

        dn-> TotFamIncW = (taxinc_r + taxinc_s) + (transinc_r+transinc_s) +
YearlyReturn*totwealth_f;


/* compute family's SE status indicator, YrWorth_f */

choosing one of the formulae below */

YrWorth_f=((taxinc_r + taxinc_s) + (transinc_r+transinc_s) +
YearlyReturn*totwealth_f);


/* NOTE that other SE status indicators can be chosen (by removing // in the
various specifications below) */

// YrWorth_f=((taxinc_r + taxinc_s) + (transinc_r+transinc_s) +
YearlyReturn*totwealth_f)/Factor;

// YrWorth_f=((taxinc_r + taxinc_s) + (transinc_r+transinc_s))/Factor;

//     YrWorth_f=((taxinc_r + taxinc_s) + (transinc_r+transinc_s));

// YrWorth_f=(taxinc_r + taxinc_s);

// YrWorth_f=(taxinc_r + taxinc_s) + YearlyReturn*totwealth_f;
```

```
/* permanently store the number of persons in family during the current year
simulation */
                    dn-> FamSize = NumFam;
        }

/* give same SE status to all family members */

        if (dn->relpos == FP_REF)

            {
                    dn-> SES_status = YrWorth_f; /* to family head */


                    if (sp != NULL)
                    {

                    sp->SES_status = YrWorth_f; /* to spouse, if exists */
                    }

                    if (nkids > 0)        /* to dependent children if exist */

                    do
                    {
                    if (kid->relpos == FP_DEP_CHILD)

                            kid-> SES_status = YrWorth_f;

                    } while ((kid=kid->rel) != head);
            }
```

/* compute SE status of non-dependent children living with family. NOTE that

these have their own incomes and wealth and are treated as a single person

family. Also NOTE that, although not reproduced below, the above choice of SE

status specification is also available to non-dependent children */

```
            if ((dn->relpos == FP_NDEP_CHILD)                {

            taxinc_r = dn->my.taxinc;

            transinc_r = dn->my.transinc;

            totwealth_f = dn->my.totwealth;
```

```
                    NumFam = 1;

                    Factor = 1;

dn->TotFamIncW = (taxinc_r + taxinc_s) + (transinc_r+transinc_s) +

YearlyReturn*totwealth_f;



                    dn-> SES_status = YrWorth_f;
          }

     } while ((dn = wctrl_next(world,dn)) != NULL);


//****************************************************************************
// Creates an array with SES_status as variable and sorts this array. Divides
// population into five equal parts and allocates SES quintile 0 to the  fifth
// of the population with lowest SES_status, etc (with quintile 4 to the group
// with highest SES status).
//****************************************************************************

dn = wctrl_first(world);                    /* go to first person */

     printf("\nStarting SES Quintile Computation\n");

  do
       {
        counter++;  /* counts number of persons in population at that time */

        } while ((dn = wctrl_next(world,dn)) != NULL);

            TotPop = counter;  /* stores population size in TotPop */

/* Create array with SES_status as variable */

     n = 0;

     dn = wctrl_first(world);

     do
```

```
        {
                heads[n] = dn-> SES_status;
                n++;

        } while ((dn = wctrl_next(world,dn)) != NULL);

/* sort SES_status array, using the Library routine 'qsort' */

        qsort (heads, TotPop, sizeof(long), compare);

        QuintSize = TotPop / 5;     /*number of persons in each quintile */

/* work out SES_status cut-off values by quintile of the population */

                CutOff0 = heads[QuintSize];

                CutOff1 = heads[2*QuintSize];

                CutOff2 = heads[3*QuintSize];

                CutOff3 = heads[4*QuintSize];

/* assign SES quintile value to each person in the population */

        dn = wctrl_first(world);

        do
        {
                if (dn->SES_status <= CutOff0)
                {
                        dn-> SES_index = 0;
                }
                else if (dn->SES_status <= CutOff1)
                {
                        dn-> SES_index = 1;
                }
                else if (dn->SES_status <= CutOff2)
                {
                        dn-> SES_index = 2;
                }
                else if (dn->SES_status <= CutOff3)
                {
                        dn-> SES_index = 3;
                }
                else if (dn->SES_status > CutOff3)
                {
```

```
                    dn-> SES_index = 4;
          }
```

/* if there is a spouse, place his_her person ID into 'spouse' */

```
               if (dn->spouse[LV] != NULL)
                    spouse = dn->spouse[LV]->pid;

               else if (dn->spouse[LV] == NULL)

                    spouse = 9999;
```

/* store people's SES_index at age 55 in 'SES_index55' and allocate to all over 55-s the SES_index the had at age 55*/

```
if (age == 55)

dn->SES_index55 = dn->SES_index;

dn = wctrl_first(world);                    /* go to first person */

     do
       {
               age = agenow(dn);   /* place person's current age into 'age' */

          if (age >= 55)
            dn->SES_index55 = dn->SES_index;

               else if (age < 55)

               dn->SES_index55 = 9999;

     } while ((dn = wctrl_next(world,dn)) != NULL);

}

   }
  }
 }   /* end of 'start in 1987' loop */
 }     /* end of SES function */
```

/************************ Compare *****************************/

/* compare function needed when using qsort */

```
int compare(void *vp, void *vq)
{
      long *p = vp, *q = vq, x;

      x = *p - *q;
      return ((x == 0.0) ? 0 : (x < 0.0) ? -1 : +1);
}
```

/******************** Computes number of kids **************************** /

```
int nkids_SES ( Dynanode *dn )
{
  Dynanode  *head,
                    *kid;
      int           nkids;

      nkids= 0;
      head = dn;
      kid = dn;
      do
      {
            if ((kid->relpos) == FP_DEP_CHILD)
            {
                  nkids++;
            }
      } while ((kid=kid->rel) != head);
  return nkids;
}
```

//******************** End Module   ****************************

The C program then writes the socio-economic status indicator to the history file and goes to the next sub-routine.

 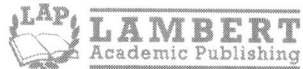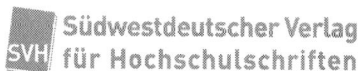

Printed in Great Britain
by Amazon